PRETERM
PRELABOUR
AMNIORRHEXIS

FRONTIERS IN FETAL MEDICINE SERIES

SERIES EDITOR: K.H. NICOLAIDES

PRETERM
PRELABOUR
AMNIORRHEXIS

S.G. CARROLL, N.J. SEBIRE AND K.H. NICOLAIDES

Harris Birthright Research Centre for Fetal Medicine
King's College Hospital Medical School
London, UK

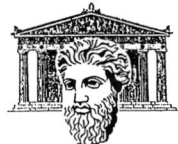

The Parthenon Publishing Group
International Publishers in Medicine, Science & Technology

NEW YORK   LONDON

The royalties from this book will be donated to the
Fetal Medicine Foundation

British Library Cataloguing in Publication Data
Carroll, S.G.
  Preterm Prelabour Amniorrhexis
  – (Frontiers in Fetal Medicine
  Series)
  I. Title II. Series
  618.32

ISBN 1-85070-692-1

Library of Congress Cataloging-in-Publication Data
Carroll, S.G. (Stephen Gerald), 1960–
Preterm prelabour amniorrhexis /
S.G. Carroll, N.J. Sebire and K.H.
Nicolaides
  p. cm. – (Frontiers in fetal
  medicine series)
Includes bibliographical references
and index.
ISBN 1-85070-692-1
1. Fetal membranes–Rupture.
2. Pregnancy– Complications.
3. Labor, Premature– Etiology.
I. Sebire, N.J. (Neil James), 1968–. II.
Nicolaides, K.H. III. Title.
IV. Series.
(DNLM. 1. Labor,
Premature–etiology. 2. Labor,
Premature–therapy. 3. Pregnancy
Complications, Infectious. 4. Fetal
Membranes, Premature Rupture.
5. Amnion. WQ 330 C319p 1995]
RG572.C37 1995
618.3'97–dc20
DNLM/DLC
for Library of Congress   95-1596
                                        CIP
                                        Rev

Published in the UK and Europe by
The Parthenon Publishing Group Ltd
Casterton Hall, Carnforth
Lancs. LA6 2LA, UK

Published in North America by
The Parthenon Publishing Group Inc,
One Blue Hill Plaza
Pearl River
New York 10965, USA

Copyright © 1996 Professor K. H.
Nicolaides

First published 1996

Composed by AMA Graphics Ltd

Printed and bound by Bookcraft
(Bath) Ltd., Midsomer Norton, UK

Contents

Acknowledgements

The authors thank the authors and publishers of the following articles for their kind permission to reproduce figures in this book.

Katz, K, Newman RB, Gill PJ. Assessment of uterine activity in ambulatory patients at high risk of preterm labor and delivery. Am J Obstet Gynecol 1986; 154: 46.

Catalano PM, Ashikaga T, Mann LI. Cervical change and uterine activity as predictors of preterm delivery. Am J Perinatol 1989; 6: 188.

Murakawa H, Utumi T, Hasegawa I, Tanaka K, Fuzimori R. Evaluation of threatened preterm delivery by transcervical ultrasonographic measurement of cervical length. Obstet Gynecol 1993; 82: 830.

Preterm delivery: incidence and complications, causes and prevention

OVERVIEW

Delivery before 37 completed weeks of gestation occurs in less than 10% of pregnancies but accounts for more than 60% of all neonatal deaths. Approximately one third of preterm deliveries are associated with preterm prelabour amniorrhexis.

This chapter examines the incidence and outcome of preterm births as well as the factors that place somebody at risk of this pregnancy complication and evaluates attempts at prediction and prevention of preterm labour.

PRETERM DELIVERY

Incidence

The reported incidence of preterm birth varies from as high as 11% to as low as 4% (Table 1.1). The disparity of incidence between the various studies presumably reflects differences in the populations examined. For example, Rush *et al* (1978), who reported an incidence of 11%, studied a socioeconomically deprived black population in South Africa, whereas Heinonen *et al* (1988) examined a more affluent, mainly caucasian population in Finland and found the incidence to be 4%.

Table 1.1. Studies reporting on the incidence of preterm delivery.

Author	N	Preterm	Study population
Heinonen *et al* 1988	31,778	4.2%	Kuopio, Finland
McGregor *et al* 1990a	202	4.5%	Denver, USA
Rush *et al* 1976	9,458	5.1%	Oxford, England
McKenzie *et al* 1994	2,139	6.8%	Dundee, Scotland
Hobel *et al* 1994	2,654	7.6%	Los Angeles, USA
Lyon *et al* 1994	11,046	8.1%	London, England
Tucker *et al* 1991	13,119	11.0%	Alabama, USA
Rush *et al* 1978	21,064	11.1%	Cape Town, South Africa
Total	**91,460**	**7.5%**	

In the United States of America, with approximately four million live singleton births per year, the overall incidence of preterm deliveries is nearly 10% (Table 1.2).

Table 1.2. Gestation at delivery of 3,891,440 singleton live births during 1989 in the United States of America (Department of Health, USA 1993).

Gestation	N	Incidence
<28 wks	23,766	0.6%
28-31 wks	42,788	1.1%
32-36 wks	310,927	8.0%
37-41 wks	3,038,496	78.1%
>41 wks	475,463	12.2%

It is impossible to determine accurately whether the incidence of preterm delivery has changed over the years because until recently prematurity was defined by a birth weight of less than 2,500 g rather than gestation at delivery. On the assumption that the vast majority of small babies are preterm, the data from the Department of Health in the United Kingdom indicate that the incidence of live births with a birth weight below 2,500 g, which is about 6–7%, has remained more or less the same since 1953, when accurate records began (Figure 1.1).

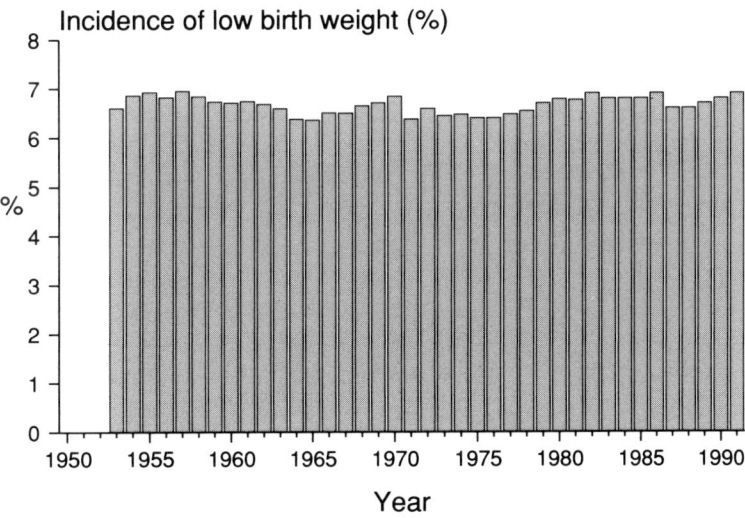

Figure 1.1. Percentage of live births with birth weight less than 2,500 g in England and Wales from 1953 to 1991 (Department of Health, UK, 1993).

Mortality and handicap

Traditionally death certificates included only the final cause of death, rather than any contributing factors, and consequently infant mortality statistics have underestimated the true contribution of prematurity (Carver *et al* 1993). However, in the United Kingdom the death certificate has recently been altered to include underlying factors as well as the direct cause of death. From these data, prematurity is implicated as a cause of death in more than 60% of all neonatal deaths and in around 85% of those with a birth weight of less than 2,500 g (Table 1.3, OPCS 1991).

Table 1.3. Causes of neonatal death in England and Wales for all births and those with birth weight less than 2,500 g (OPCS 1991).

Cause of neonatal death	All weights	<2,500 g
Prematurity	62%	84%
Congenital anomalies	29%	22%
Non infectious respiratory disease	24%	29%
Intrauterine hypoxia	8%	4%
Infection	6%	5%
Haemolytic disease of the newborn	<1%	<1%

The antenatal management and timing of obstetric interventions in all high risk pregnancies, and particularly in those with threatened preterm delivery or preterm prelabour amniorrhexis, necessitate accurate knowledge of current postnatal survival statistics. In a study where obstetricians were requested to make decisions on the management of high risk pregnancies, management was primarily dependent on the obstetricians', perception of postnatal survival, but their perceived rates varied widely (Goldenberg *et al* 1982).

Gestation and birth weight

Survival of preterm infants is mainly dependent on gestation at delivery and birth weight. Survival increases from less than 10% before 24 weeks to 90% by 30 weeks (Figure 1.2). Similarly, survival increases with birth weight from about 10% at 500 g to over 90% at 1,500 g (Figure 1.3).

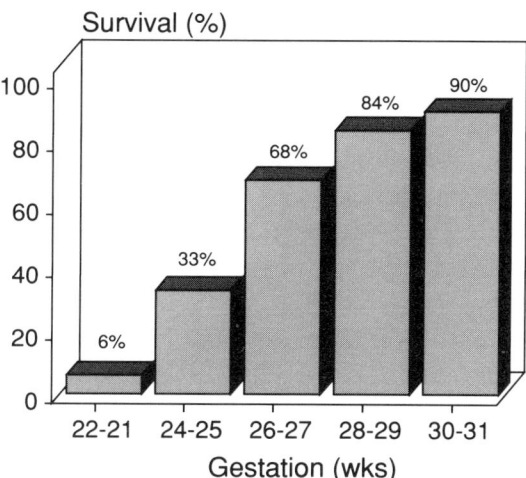

Figure 1.2. Postnatal survival of live born infants according to gestational age at delivery. The data are derived from nine major recent studies on a total of 12,866 live born infants delivered at 22-31 weeks (Hack & Fanaroff 1989, Wood *et al* 1989, Ferrara *et al* 1989, Kilbride *et al* 1990, Working Group on the Very Low Birth Weight Infant 1990, Hack *et al* 1991, Phelps *et al* 1991, Copper *et al* 1993, Whyte *et al* 1993).

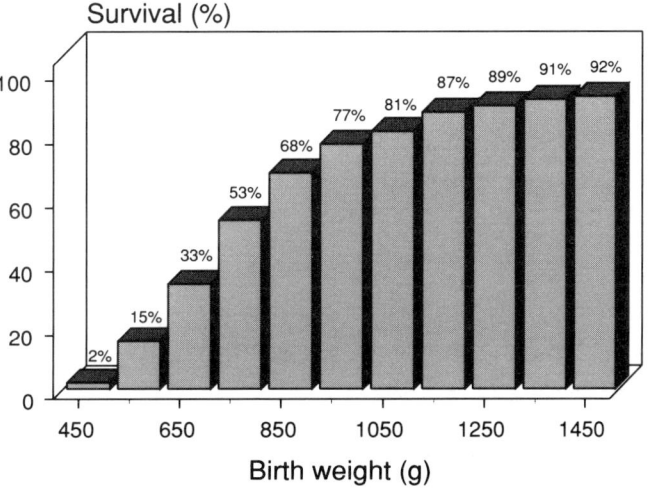

Figure 1.3. Postnatal survival of live born infants according to birth weight. The data are derived from 14 major recent studies on a total of 26,064 live born infants delivered with birth weight of less than 1,500 g (Hack & Fanaroff 1989, Wood *et al* 1989, Powers *et al* 1989, Resnick *et al* 1989, Kilbride *et al* 1990, Working Group on the Very Low Birth Weight Infant 1990, Vermont-Oxford Trials Network Database Project 1990, Victorian Infant Collaborative Study Group 1991, Hack *et al* 1991, Phelps *et al* 1991, Alberman & Botting 1991, Copper *et al* 1993, Whyte *et al* 1993, Howell & Vert 1993).

On the basis of the data on survival by gestation (Figure 1.2) and birth weight (Figure 1.3), it is recommended that infants born after 24 weeks should receive full resuscitation, whereas for those born at less than 24 weeks and weighing less than 500 g only comfort care should be given (Hack & Fanaroff 1993, Allen *et al* 1993).

Neonatal care

In addition to gestation at delivery and birth weight, survival is also dependent on rapidly improving facilities for neonatal care, and this can account for the variation in survival between centres. Furthermore, improved survival of the very premature infant has been achieved without an increase in the rate of handicap among survivors. This is illustrated by data from centres reporting survival and handicap in their current practice compared to that five to eight years previously (Table 1.4). For example, Kilbride *et al* (1990) reported that, in very preterm infants with a birth weight of 800 g or less, neonatal survival increased from 14% in 1982 to 40% in 1985; the rate of handicap among survivors was reduced from 67% to 13%. Similarly, the incidence of cerebral haemorrhage has not increased with increasing survival. Cooke (1991) reported that between 1980 and 1990 the survival rate for babies born before 35 weeks increased by 56%, but the incidence of cerebral haemorrhage remained unchanged at around 40%.

Table 1.4. Studies comparing survival and handicap of very preterm infants from the same centres at around 1980 and five to eight years later. In three of the four series there was a major improvement in survival and this was achieved with a simultaneous decrease in handicap. BW = mean birth weight.

Author	Criterion	N	Year	BW	Survival	Handicap
Hack & Fanaroff 1989	<750 g	98	1982	567 g	20%	same
		129	1988	551 g	18%	same
Ferrara *et al* 1989	<750 g	40	1981	713 g	21%	23%
		71	1987	676 g	53%	22%
Kilbride *et al* 1990	<801 g	63	1980	*	14%	67%
		149	1985	670 g	40%	13%
Kitchen *et al* 1991	<1000 g	351	1979	-	25%	51%
		560	1987	-	38%	30%

* The paper states that the birth weight was not significantly different from 670 g

In three of the four studies summarised in Table 1.4, survival increased and the handicap rate was reduced over a period of five to eight years. Although in the study of Hack and Fanaroff (1989) there was no overall improvement in survival, when the data were analysed according to gestational age, survival of infants born at 25-27 weeks improved from 52% in 1982 to 71% in 1988. A review of follow up studies of very low birth weight infants (less than 1,500 g), also concluded that during the last 30 years survival has improved dramatically whereas the median incidence of disability in survivors has decreased from around 30% to 20% (Escobar *et al* 1991).

A major recent advance in neonatal care has been the introduction of surfactant therapy, which has been shown to decrease substantially the risk of death and other associated complications of respiratory distress syndrome. A study of 4,193 neonates with a birth weight of 600-1,300 g compared outcome after the introduction of surfactant therapy with historical controls and reported an 8% decrease in mortality (Horbar *et al* 1993). A randomised study of 310 infants born at 23-26 weeks reported that surfactant treatment, compared to placebo, was associated with an 18% increase in survival and a two-fold reduction in pulmonary haemorrhage (Ferrara *et al* 1994). Furthermore, follow up data have demonstrated that surfactant increased survival without increasing the proportion of infants with neurological or respiratory impairments (Ferrera *et al* 1994, Gunkel *et al* 1994).

The beneficial effects of maternal corticosteroids and surfactant therapy are additive. In a multicenter randomised study of 188 infants born at less than 32 weeks of gestation, the incidence of intraventricular haemorrhage was 10% in the group that received maternal corticosteroid plus surfactant, compared to 48% in the placebo and surfactant group (Kari *et al* 1994).

PRELABOUR AMNIORRHEXIS

Contribution to preterm delivery

Preterm prelabour amniorrhexis complicates about one third of preterm deliveries (Table 1.5).

Table 1.5. Studies reporting on preterm prelabour amniorrhexis as a percentage of preterm deliveries. In a total of 30,272 preterm deliveries, 29% were associated with preterm prelabour amniorrhexis.

Author	N	Preterm delivery
Kaltreider & Kohl 1980	11,832	34%
Naeye & Peters 1980	6,613	32%
Johnson *et al* 1981	1,174	38%
Daikoku *et al* 1982	477	43%
Main *et al* 1985	534	40%
Meis *et al* 1987a	206	39%
Goldenberg *et al* 1990	7,991	18%
Tucker *et al* 1991	1,445	28%
Total	**30,272**	**29%**

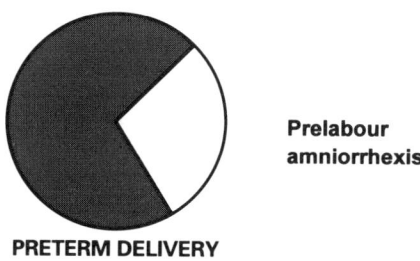

Prelabour amniorrhexis

PRETERM DELIVERY

Mortality and handicap

In pregnancies complicated by preterm prelabour amniorrhexis there are essentially three causes of neonatal death: prematurity, sepsis and pulmonary hypoplasia. However, several studies have reported that the overall survival of preterm infants delivered after prelabour amniorrhexis is not significantly different from those delivered at the same gestation after labour with intact membranes (Hack *et al* 1991, Varner & Galask 1981, Daikoku *et al* 1981, Owen *et al* 1990a, Wolf *et al* 1993, Shennan *et al* 1985). Therefore, the major risk of preterm prelabour amniorrhexis is the progression to preterm delivery and its associated complications such as respiratory distress syndrome (Schreiber & Benedetti 1980, Morales 1987, Van Reempts *et al* 1993).

The findings of the above studies are in apparent contradiction to those from studies reporting that a high proportion of deaths in pregnancies with preterm prelabour amniorrhexis are due to pulmonary hypoplasia (see Table 1.7). In addition, studies examining the consequences of chorioamnionitis in pregnancies with preterm amniorrhexis have reported that perinatal mortality is higher in the presence rather than absence of infection (Garite & Freeman 1982, Morales 1987).

Culture of fetal blood samples obtained by cordocentesis in pregnancies complicated by preterm prelabour amniorrhexis has demonstrated that, in the presence of fetal bacteraemia, spontaneous delivery occurs within a few days of amniorrhexis (see Chapter 2). Therefore, in infected cases, survival is primarily dependent on gestation at delivery and also the severity of the neonatal sepsis. The risk of infection is inversely proportional to the gestation at amniorrhexis (see Chapter 2) but the importance of infection on adverse pregnancy outcome is underestimated because currently available data are primarily derived from tertiary referral centres; patients with intrauterine infection, especially at less than 24 weeks of gestation, are unlikely to be referred to tertiary centres for further assessment because in these cases there is spontaneous abortion soon after amniorrhexis. Another factor that causes underestimation of the importance of infection is that the vast majority of preterm births occur after 32 weeks (see Table 1.2) and survival in this group is high, irrespective of the presence or absence of sepsis.

In pregnancies with no evidence of infection, the interval between amniorrhexis and delivery may be several months (see Chapter 2); in these cases there are two major causes of neonatal death, pulmonary hypoplasia and severe prematurity. As with infection, the adverse consequences of pulmonary hypoplasia are underestimated in studies reporting on overall survival of pregnancies with preterm prelabour amniorrhexis because, in the vast majority of cases, amniorrhexis and delivery occur after 27 weeks (see Table 1.2) and in this group there is no risk of pulmonary hypoplasia. In addition, until recently, pregnancies with amniorrhexis at less than 24 weeks (the very group at high risk of pulmonary hypoplasia) were usually terminated because of the fears of infectious complications for the mother.

Recent studies on the outcome of neonates from pregnancies with prelabour amniorrhexis that were managed expectantly have reported that the risk of neonatal death is related to the gestation at amniorrhexis and decreases from 66% for those with amniorrhexis before 20 weeks to less than 10% when amniorrhexis occurs after 26 weeks (Table 1.6).

Table 1.6. Incidence of postnatal death in live births from pregnancies complicated by preterm prelabour amniorrhexis according to gestational age (weeks) at amniorrhexis. The total results are also illustrated in the figure below.

Author	N	Incidence of postnatal death by gestation at amniorrhexis (weeks)			
		<20	**20-24**	**25-26**	**27-28**
Taylor & Garite 1984	44	50%	75%	65%	-
Beydoun & Yasin 1986	54	-	45%	24%	14%
Moretti & Sibai 1988	107	86%	78%	37%	-
Major & Kitzmiller 1990	60	-	24%	8%	-
Morales & Talley 1993	78	87%	46%	-	
Carroll et al 1995	100	50%	37%	10%	4%
Total	**443**	**66%**	**50%**	**33%**	**7%**

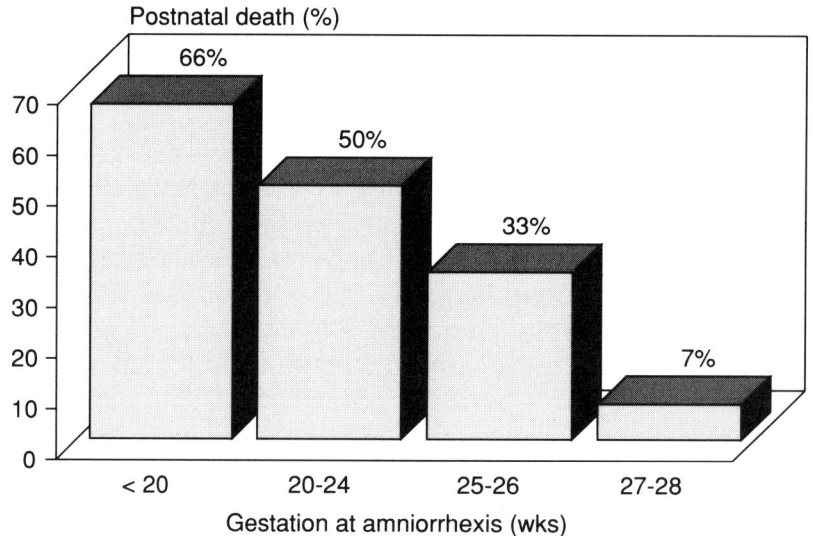

In addition to gestation at amniorrhexis, the risk of postnatal death is also related to the gestation at delivery. In a study of 172 pregnancies with preterm prelabour amniorrhexis at 12-36

weeks of gestation that resulted in livebirths, postnatal death decreased from 43% for those that were born at 24-28 weeks, to 13% for those born at 29-32 weeks and 4% for those born after 32 weeks (Figure 1.4).

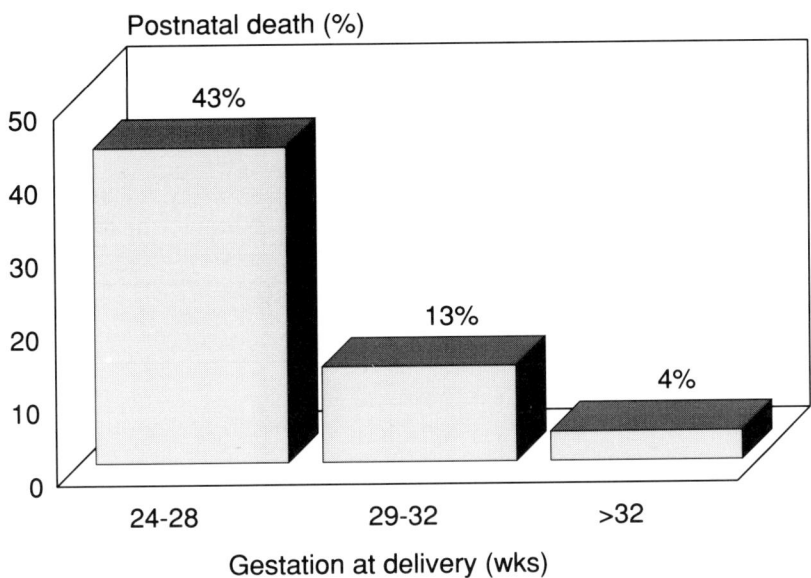

Figure 1.4. Incidence of postnatal death in livebirths from pregnancies complicated by preterm prelabour amniorrhexis according to gestation at delivery (Carroll *et al* 1995).

In the studies of pregnancies with prelabour amniorrhexis that were managed expectantly and resulted in livebirths, there were two causes of postnatal death, pulmonary hypoplasia and prematurity-related complications. The incidence of postnatal death due to pulmonary hypoplasia in live births was primarily related to the gestation at amniorrhexis, rather than at delivery, and decreased from approximately 50% for those with amniorrhexis before 20 weeks, to 20% for those with amniorrhexis at 20-24 weeks and less than 5% for amniorrhexis after 24 weeks (Table 1.7).

In contrast, death due to prematurity-related complications is primarily dependent on the gestation at delivery (Carroll *et al* 1995), and the incidence is similar to that of all preterm deliveries (see Figure 1.2).

Table 1.7. Incidence of postnatal deaths due to pulmonary hypoplasia in live births from pregnancies complicated by preterm prelabour amniorrhexis according to gestational age at amniorrhexis. The total results are also demonstrated in the figure below.

Author	Death due to pulmonary hypoplasia by gestation at amniorrhexis					
	<20 weeks		20-24 weeks		25-28 weeks	
	N	Death	N	Death	N	Death
Nimrod *et al* 1984	5	40%	15	27%	27	4%
Blott & Greenough 1988	14	50%	7	14%	9	0%
Rotschild *et al* 1990	8	63%	19	37%	50	8%
Carroll *et al* 1995	22	50%	46	15%	32	0%
Total	**49**	**51%**	**87**	**22%**	**118**	**3%**

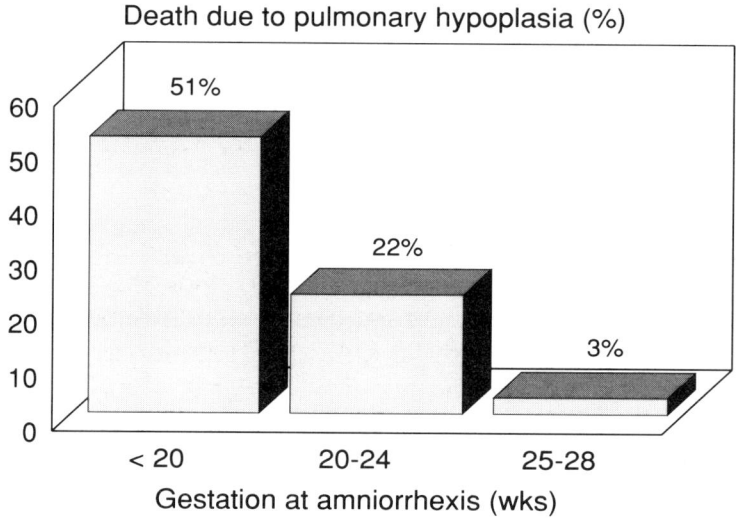

Death due to pulmonary hypoplasia (%)

Gestation at amniorrhexis (wks)

The findings that the risk of pulmonary hypoplasia is inversely related to the gestation at amniorrhexis and that pulmonary hypoplasia is unlikely if amniorrhexis occurs after 24 weeks, irrespective of the interval between amniorrhexis and delivery, are compatible with current knowledge on lung development. Animal studies involving chronic drainage of amniotic fluid have demonstrated that oligohydramnios interferes with lung development (Collins *et al* 1986, Moessinger *et al* 1986). The magnitude of this interference depends mainly on the time of onset rather than the duration of oligohydramnios. Maximum interference is observed when oligohydramnios is present during the canalicular phase of lung development, which in the human is at 16-24 weeks of gestation (Moessinger *et al* 1986).

Long term prognosis of infants from pregnancies with amniorrhexis is primarily dependent on gestation at delivery. The overall incidence of permanent neurological handicap in infants born prematurely after prelabour amniorrhexis is not higher than in infants born at the same gestation due to other causes. In a follow up study of 383 infants born at 26-34 weeks of gestation, the incidence of handicap at one year of age in those born after prelabour amniorrhexis was not significantly different from those with idiopathic prematurity (Shennan *et al* 1985).

In contrast to overall outcome of pregnancies with amniorrhexis, infants from pregnancies with clinical chorioamnionitis may have developmental delay. In a follow up study of 106 infants delivered before 37 weeks of gestation, at one year of age the incidence of a low developmental index score (less than 85/100) was significantly higher in the cases where preterm delivery was associated with clinical chorioamnionitis (Hardt *et al* 1985).

A study of 127 preterm infants who were screened by neonatal cranial ultrasound examinations reported that the incidence of white matter necrosis and periventricular leukomalacia, found in 18% of the cases, was related to both the gestation at delivery and the presence of purulent amniotic fluid (Bejar *et al* 1988).

Long term pulmonary function in infants born after preterm prelabour amniorrhexis may be normal; in a longitudinal study of 22 such infants, serial functional residual capacity measurements were carried out until the age of two years and these were not significantly different from normal controls (Thompson *et al* 1990).

RISK FACTORS FOR PRETERM DELIVERY

Risk scoring systems

Scoring systems have been developed with the aim of identifying the women likely to deliver prematurely so that preventive measures can be undertaken. The scoring systems are primarily based on variables from the social and past obstetric history of the women as well as their daily habits and certain features in their current pregnancy. The most widely used system is that of Creasy *et al* (1980), which is summarised in Table 1.8.

In a study of 966 pregnancies, the patients were allocated a risk score at their first antenatal clinic visit; the high risk group (score $\geq$10), which comprised 9% of the total, contained 44% of all preterm deliveries (Creasy *et al* 1980).

In eight studies involving a total of 25,842 pregnancies, 16% received a high risk score but this group contained only 37% of the preterm deliveries (Table 1.9). Risk scoring is even less useful in primigravidae, because past obstetric history is the most important factor in the scoring system (Mueller-Heubach and Guzick 1989).

Table 1.9. Studies examining the value of risk scoring in the prediction of preterm delivery. In the total of 25,842 pregnancies, 16% had a high score and this group identified 37% of the preterm deliveries that occurred in 9.8% of the cases.

Author	N	High score	Preterm delivery	
			Total	Sensitivity
Creasy *et al* 1980	966	9%	5.6%	44%
Herron *et al* 1982*	1,150	10%	4.7%	56%
Guzick *et al* 1984	2,865	24%	8.8%	62%
Main *et al* 1985	534	29%	16.3%	48%
Mueller-Heubach & Guzick 1989	4,591	18%	10.1%	40%
Owen *et al* 1990b	7,478	15%	12.1%	29%
Goldenberg *et al* 1990	7,991	19%	8.5%	35%
Guinn *et al* 1994	267	4%	9.8%	15%
Total	**25,842**	**16%**	**9.8%**	37%

* In this study results were not given for preterm delivery but for preterm labour

Ethnic group

In Western societies the incidence of preterm delivery is higher in all ethnic minorities but particularly in those of Afro-Caribbean origin. However, It is likely that the underlying mechanism for ethnic differences is environmental, such as nutrition, health behaviour, educational standards and utilisation of antenatal care, rather than genetic predisposition (Virji & Cottington 1991). A study of 8,903 women in Boston, USA, reported that when social

Table 1.8. Risk scoring system. Each feature (*) receives points and a total score of at least 10 is thought to identify a group at high risk for preterm birth. Adapted from Creasy *et al* (1980).

Points	Feature	Parameter
1	Demographic	*Low socioeconomic status
	Past history	*One abortion
		*Less than one year since last birth
	Daily habits	*Work outside home
	This pregnancy	*Unusual fatigue
2	Demographic	*Single parent
		*Age less than 20 or more than 40 years
	Past history	*Two abortions
	Daily habits	*More than 10 cigarettes per day
	This pregnancy	*Weight gain by 32 weeks less than 13 kg
		*Albuminuria
		*Bacteriuria
		*Hypertension
3	Demographic	*Very low socioeconomic status
		*Height less than 150 cm
		*Weight less than 45 kg
	Past history	*Three abortions
	Daily habits	*Heavy work
		*Long tiring trip
	This pregnancy	*Breech presentation at 32 weeks
		*Weight loss of more than 2 kg
		*Engagement of the fetal head
		*Febrile illness
4	Demographic	*Age less than 18 years
	Past history	*Pyelonephritis
	This pregnancy	*Vaginal bleed after 12 weeks
		*Cervical effacement or dilatation
		*Uterine irritability
5	Past history	*Uterine anomaly
		*Second trimester loss
	This pregnancy	*Placenta praevia
		*Polyhydramnios
10	Past history	*Preterm delivery
		*Second trimester losses
	This pregnancy	*Multiple pregnancy
		*Abdominal operation

and demographic factors, including age less than 20 years, single marital status, receiving welfare support and not having graduated from high school were accounted for, maternal race was no longer a significant risk factor for preterm delivery (Lieberman *et al* 1987). Similarly, a study of 7,478 women in Alabama, USA, reported that race does not predict preterm delivery if other factors are adjusted for (Owen *et al* 1990b).

Maternal age

The incidence of preterm delivery is highest in women aged under 20 and over 35 years. The risk of poorer pregnancy outcome in teenagers is reported in most studies but this risk is probably due to associated social and behavioural factors rather than intrinsic biological determinants of the young age (Zuckerman *et al* 1984).

For women over the age of 35 years there is controversy whether the apparently increased risk is due to their age (Lehmann & Chism 1987), or other confounding factors such as preexisting medical disorders and complications of pregnancy leading to iatrogenic preterm delivery (Kirz *et al* 1985, Aldous & Edmonson 1993).

Maternal size

Low prepregnancy maternal weight is associated with an increased chance of preterm delivery, particularly in women who are very underweight (less than 80% of recommended weight for height) and have low weight gain during pregnancy (Mitchell & Lerner 1989). Furthermore, maternal underweight may act synergistically with the other risk factors (Nandi & Nelson 1992). Maternal obesity is not associated with an increased incidence of preterm delivery, but infants of obese mothers who are born prematurely have a worse neonatal survival for gestational age, probably due to the 'diabetes-like' metabolic milieu of such pregnancies (Lucas *et al* 1988).

Maternal employment, exercise and psychological stress

A study based on 20,613 married women with singleton pregnancies in Wales reported that the proportion of deliveries which were preterm was no higher in those who were employed than in the unemployed group; it was recommended that healthy women can safely continue in employment during pregnancy (Murphy *et al* 1984). A study of more than 250,000 live births in Scotland reported that there was a small increase in risk for preterm delivery in women who had manual rather than non-manual jobs, and the risk was particularly high for electrical and metal workers (Sanjose *et al* 1991).

Prospective studies regarding physical activity in pregnancy have reported that neither heavy work nor exercise are associated with preterm delivery but prolonged periods of standing (more than eight hours per day) may be associated with a small (1.3 fold) increase in risk (Klebanoff *et al* 1990).

A prospective study of 8,719 pregnancies examined the effect of psychological stress and reported that high levels of stress in the third trimester were associated with an increased likelihood of preterm delivery; stress before or during the early stages of pregnancy had no adverse effects (Hedegaard *et al* 1993).

Cigarette smoking

The incidence of preterm delivery is higher in women that smoke than in non-smokers (Wen *et al* 1990). It has been suggested that smoking may induce labour by increasing the amniotic fluid concentration of the inflammatory mediator platelet activating factor; cigarette smoke is a potent inhibitor of the enzyme that degrades platelet activating factor (Narahara & Johnston 1993).

Drug abuse

There is an association between drug abuse and preterm delivery (Heffner *et al* 1993). The risk is particularly high with cocaine (Spence *et al* 1991), which may act through its effect on placental production of prostaglandins (Monga *et al* 1994). A study of cocaine abusers reported that on average the length of gestation was reduced by two weeks compared to matched controls (McGregor *et al* 1987). The highest risk is with 'crack' cocaine that is associated with a greater than three-fold increase in the proportion of preterm deliveries, compared to controls (Cherukuri *et al* 1988). Marijuana use in pregnant women is associated with a small reduction in birth weight but has no effect on the length of gestation (Zuckerman *et al* 1989).

Parity and inter-pregnancy interval

The incidence of preterm delivery may be slightly higher in primiparae than multiparae (Kaltreider & Kohl 1980, Heffner *et al* 1993). Although an inter-pregnancy interval of less than 18 months is associated with a lower birth weight, it has no effect on gestation length (Lieberman *et al* 1989).

Previous preterm delivery

All studies examining the importance of a history of previous preterm delivery have consistently reported a greater risk of delivering prematurely in the current pregnancy, the relative risk being 2-7 (Table 1.10).

Table 1.10. Relative risk of preterm delivery following previous preterm delivery.

Author	N	Preterm	Relative risk
Kaltreider & Kohl 1980	240,474	5%	2
Guzick *et al* 1984	2,865	9%	3
Mueller-Heubach & Guzick 1989	4,490	10%	2
Owen *et al* 1990b	7,478	9%	2
McGregor *et al* 1990b	229	8%	4
McGregor *et al* 1990a	202	5%	7
De Haas *et al* 1991	420	-	4
Heffner *et al* 1993	778	-	3
Lockwood *et al* 1993	429	11%	2
Guinn *et al* 1994	267	10%	2

Previous abortion

Data from the 1970s suggested that having had a termination of pregnancy increased the chance of subsequent preterm delivery (Kaltreider & Kohl 1980). However, several more recent studies using appropriate controls and with modern techniques of legal termination of pregnancy have found no significant relationship between either having had a termination of pregnancy or the number of terminations, and subsequent preterm delivery (Linn *et al* 1983, Ekwo *et al* 1993, De Haas *et al* 1991, Heffner *et al* 1993).

Cervical cone biopsy

Cone biopsy is associated with increased risk of preterm delivery (Heffner *et al* 1993, Kristensen *et al* 1993). Reports originally demonstrated this association after cold knife cone biopsies (Jones *et al* 1979), and it was postulated that the mode of conisation may be important. However, a recent study has shown that preterm delivery in women who have had a previous laser cone biopsy was 38% compared to 6% in normal controls (Hagen & Skjeldestad 1993).

Uterine abnormalities

A spectrum of uterine abnormalities due to abnormal fusion of the mullerian ducts or failure of absorption of the septum are thought to be present in 0.5% to 5% of deliveries (Buttram & Gibbons 1979, Golan *et al* 1989).

In three studies on a total of 627 pregnancies in 286 patients with a variety of proven uterine abnormalities, the incidence of preterm delivery was 22% and this was related to the type of uterine abnormality (Table 1.11). In addition to preterm delivery, Heinonen *et al* (1982) reported that 29% of the patients with uterine abnormalities had a miscarriage.

Table 1.11. Uterine abnormalities and incidence of preterm delivery (Heinonen *et al* 1982, Michalas 1991, Golan *et al* 1992).

Abnormality	N	Preterm delivery
Unicornuate	49	31%
Didelphic	65	31%
Bicornuate	350	24%
Septate	144	12%
Total	**627**	**22%**

Multiple pregnancy

Preterm delivery is much more common in multiple than singleton pregnancies; it occurs in nearly 50% of twin pregnancies and in around 90% of triplet pregnancies (Table 1.12 and Figure 1.5).

Table 1.12. Gestation at delivery of live births from singleton (3,891,440), twin (88,848) and triplet (2,711) pregnancies in the United States of America during 1989. (Department of Health, USA 1993).

Gestation	Singletons	Twins	Triplets
<20 wks	0.02%	0.20%	0.30%
20-27 wks	0.59%	4.52%	11.66%
28-31 wks	1.10%	6.57%	20.51%
32-36 wks	7.99%	35.69%	53.33%
37-39 wks	40.64%	40.75%	10.81%
40-41 wks	37.44%	9.15%	2.29%
≥42 wks	12.20%	3.12%	1.10%

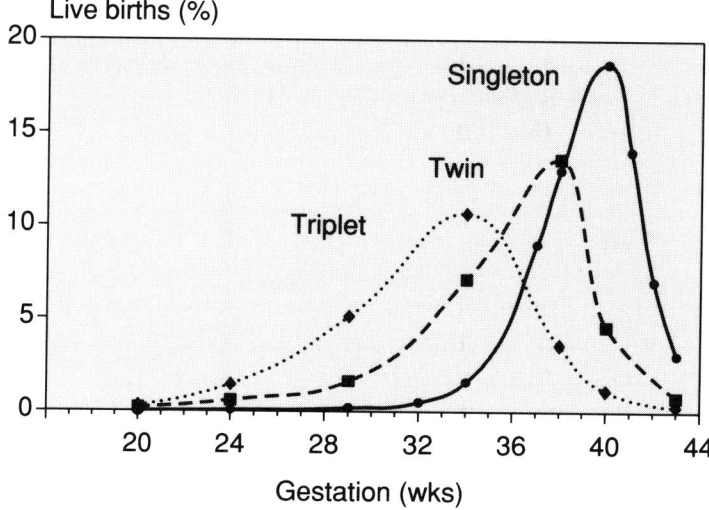

Figure 1.5. Frequency distribution of gestation at delivery for live births from singleton, twin and triplet pregnancies in the United States of America during 1989. Adapted from Department of Health, USA, 1993.

Fetal abnormalities

Certain fetal abnormalities, particularly those resulting in polyhydramnios, such as anencephaly, diaphragmatic hernia, or bowel obstruction, can cause preterm delivery.

Vaginal bleeding

Vaginal bleeding during pregnancy is associated with increased risk for preterm delivery. First trimester bleeding is associated with a two-fold increase in risk, whereas with bleeding in the second and third trimesters there is a 10-fold increase in risk (Ekwo *et al* 1992, Harger *et al* 1990, Heffner *et al* 1993).

Coitus

There is an association between a history of multiple sexual partners and preterm delivery, particularly preterm prelabour amniorrhexis (Toth *et al* 1988). However, coitus with one sexual partner is not associated with increased incidence of preterm birth with or without amniorrhexis, suggesting that it is infection secondary to sexual behaviour rather than coitus itself which causes preterm birth (Kurki & Ylikorkala 1993). The effect of coitus on a group of women at high risk for preterm delivery, those with twin gestations, was examined by a prospective study and was not reported to be associated with any significant increase in the rate of preterm delivery (Neilson & Mutambira 1989).

Uterine activity

Uterine activity is present throughout normal pregnancy. During the first 20 weeks of gestation, contractile activity is of very low intensity but thereafter until term there is a progressive increase in both the frequency and intensity of contractions (Alvarez & Caldeyro 1950).

Several studies of home uterine activity monitoring in pregnancies at high risk for preterm delivery have reported a significant increase in uterine activity 24-48 hours before the onset of preterm labour (Figure 1.6; Bell 1983, Katz *et al* 1986, Martin *et al* 1990, Garite *et al* 1990).

Similarly, a study of women, who had cervical cerclage in their current pregnancy, reported that there was a gradual increase in frequency of contractions with gestation and an abrupt rise within 24 hours before the onset of labour (Robichaux *et al* 1990). In another study of singleton, twin, triplet and quadruplet pregnancies, uterine activity was not significantly different between the groups and they all had a rise in activity within 48 hours prior to the diagnosis of labour (Garite *et al* 1990).

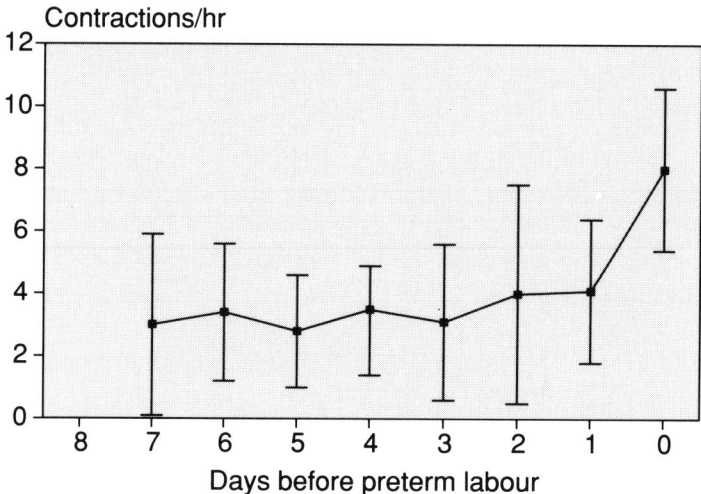

Figure 1.6. Home uterine activity monitoring in pregnancies at high risk for preterm delivery demonstrating frequency of contractions (mean and standard deviation) with an increase in mean contraction frequency within 24 hours before the onset of preterm labour. Adapted from Katz *et al* 1986 with permission.

Campbell *et al* (1991) examined 101 pregnancies with preterm prelabour amniorrhexis at 26-34 weeks; home uterine activity monitoring was performed daily until delivery. There was no increase in activity immediately following membrane rupture but, as in patients with intact membranes who deliver prematurely, there was a marked rise in contraction frequency in the 48 hours preceding the onset of preterm labour.

There are also three studies reporting that preterm labour is preceded by increased uterine activity for several weeks. Katz *et al* (1986) studied 34 pregnancies and reported that the frequency of contractions in those that delivered preterm, compared to term deliveries, was higher for several weeks before the onset of labour (Figure 1.7). Similarly, Nageotte *et al* (1988) monitored contractions from 30 weeks of gestation in 2,446 pregnancies and found that average uterine activity was greatest at any gestation in those who subsequently developed preterm labour. Morrison *et al* (1990) monitored uterine activity at 14-19 weeks of gestation in a group of 136 women at high risk for preterm delivery and reported that those who subsequently developed preterm labour had a small rise in average uterine activity from as early as 18 weeks.

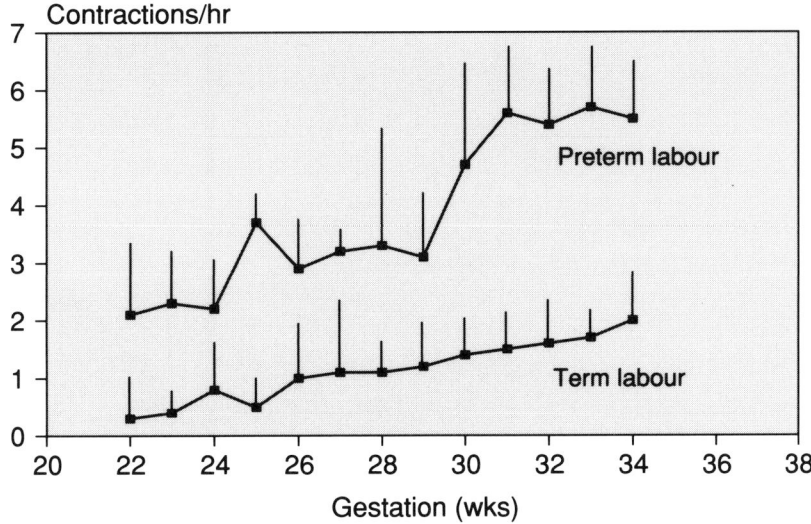

Figure 1.7. Frequency of contractions (mean and one standard deviation), during pregnancy in patients having preterm labour and patients having term labour. Adapted from Katz *et al* (1986) with permission.

Studies evaluating home monitoring of uterine activity in providing an early warning of preterm labour, compared to the development of symptoms, have reported conflicting results.

Newman *et al* (1990) examined 79 women with preterm prelabour amniorrhexis at 26-34 weeks of gestation, and found an increase in uterine activity on average 11 hours before the development of symptoms. However, the same authors found that neither objective monitoring nor maternal symptom reporting were of value in distinguishing between patients with and without cervical changes. Iams *et al* (1990) examined 51 women who presented in preterm labour and reported that those who presented because of symptoms were more likely to have cervical changes (cervix more than 2 cm dilated), compared to women who presented purely on the basis of recorded contractions. However, Martin *et al* (1990) examined 102 pregnancies at high risk for preterm delivery and showed that neither the incidence of preterm labour nor the likelihood of successful tocolysis was significantly different in patients presenting with symptoms compared to those presenting because of a recorded increase in uterine activity.

Asymptomatic bacteriuria

Asymptomatic bacteriuria (pure growth of more than 10^5 organisms per mL in a clean catch specimen of urine) occurs in around 5% of pregnancies (Kincaid-Smith & Bullen 1965, Little 1966, Patrick 1967, Carroll *et al* 1968, Gower *et al* 1968, Robertson *et al* 1968, Gruneberg *et al* 1969). In 30-50% of the cases there is subsequent development of pyelonephritis (Kincaid-Smith & Bullen 1965, Dixon & Brant 1967, Patrick 1967, Elder *et al* 1971).

Pyelonephritis, as well as other maternal febrile infections, such as pneumonia, is associated with increased rates of preterm delivery (Gilstrap *et al* 1981, Madinger *et al* 1989). Several studies have also shown that in women with asymptomatic bacteriuria the incidence of preterm delivery is twice as high as in women without bacteriuria. Thus in four studies involving a total of 6,032 pregnancies, 432 had untreated asymptomatic bacteriuria and the incidence of preterm delivery in this group was 9%, compared to 5% for controls (Table 1.13; Layton 1964, Patrick 1967, Robertson *et al* 1968, Wren 1969).

Table 1.13. Cohort studies examining the incidence of preterm delivery in the presence or absence of asymptomatic bacteriuria.

Author	N	Incidence of preterm delivery	
		Bacteriuric	**Controls**
Layton 1964	176	6%	8%
Patrick 1967	575	9%	4%
Robertson *et al* 1968	2,184	6%	3%
Wren 1969	3,099	17%	7%
Total	**6,034**	**9%**	**5%**

Abnormal cervico-vaginal flora

The incidence of preterm delivery in pregnancies with abnormal cervico-vaginal flora at the first antenatal visit is three times higher than in women with normal swabs (McGregor *et al* 1990a, Hay *et al* 1994). The link between genital tract infection and preterm prelabour amniorrhexis and preterm delivery is discussed in detail in Chapter 2.

Increased cervico-vaginal fibronectin

Fibronectins are a family of large molecular weight glycoproteins found primarily in the extracellular matrix. Using immuno-histochemical techniques, a specific type of fibronectin, bearing an oncofetal domain, is found at the chorio-decidual interface and in-vitro studies have shown that the production of fetal fibronectin by chorion cells is increased by inflammatory mediators such as interleukin and tumour necrosis factor (Jackson *et al* 1993).

The detection of fetal fibronectin in cervical and vaginal secretions may be useful in predicting preterm delivery. In a longitudinal study of 163 normal pregnancies, cervico-vaginal swabs were taken on an average of four occasions at 5-40 weeks of gestation (Lockwood *et al* 1991). A specific monoclonal antibody was used to measure fetal fibronectin and, if the level was above 50 ng/mL, the test was considered to be positive. The incidence of a positive test was about 50% before 10 weeks, decreased to a nadir of 2% by 30 weeks and rose again after 37 weeks to 30%. The assay was also performed in women who were admitted with either preterm labour with intact membranes (n=117) or preterm prelabour amniorrhexis (n=65). Fibronectin swabs were positive in 94% of those with amniorrhexis, and the mean interval from membrane rupture to delivery was 2.1 days in those with positive swabs compared to 21 days in the small group with negative swabs. Similarly, in subjects with preterm labour and intact membranes, preterm delivery occurred in 83% of those with positive swabs and in only 19% of those with a negative test (Lockwood *et al* 1991).

In a subsequent prospective study of 429 pregnancies, swabs were taken at two weekly intervals at 24-36 weeks and weekly thereafter. A positive fetal fibronectin test (more than 60 ng/mL at any visit) predicted 73% of the 47 preterm deliveries and the false positive rate was 28%; on average a positive test preceded preterm delivery by about three weeks (Lockwood *et al* 1993). In a similar study of 87 women with a high risk score for preterm delivery, weekly swabs for fibronectin were performed at 24-34 weeks of gestation; a positive test (more than 50 ng/mL at any visit) predicted 92% of the 27 preterm deliveries but the false positive rate was 47% (Nageotte *et al* 1994).

These findings suggest that fibronectin determinations may provide useful prediction of preterm delivery but more widespread application would necessitate modifications to the test to reduce the false positive rate.

High vaginal pH

In normal pregnancy the vaginal fluid is acidic (pH less than 4) because of the presence of lactobacilli which convert glycogen to lactic acid. In a study of women in preterm labour with intact membranes and preterm prelabour amniorrhexis, vaginal pH was significantly increased and this was thought to be the consequence of change in vaginal flora (Riedewald *et al* 1990).

In a prospective study of 115 women with a high risk score for preterm delivery, the vaginal pH was measured at weekly intervals from 23 weeks of gestation (Ernest *et al* 1989). The test was abnormal (mean pH of all measurements more than 4.5) in 24% of the patients and in this group the incidence of preterm prelabour amniorrhexis was three times higher than in those with normal pH (32% versus 10%); However, if the data were to be used prospectively (any pH value above 4.5), the positive predictive value of an abnormal pH would have been only 19%.

Cervical assessment

The cervix is composed of collagenous connective tissue, smooth muscle and ground substance. During pregnancy, probably under the influence of oestrogen, the cervix changes from a firm inelastic organ to a soft, highly distensible and elastic one. However, a multicentre randomised controlled trial, on a total of 5,602 pregnancies, reported that routine cervical examinations at every prenatal visit are not useful (Buekens *et al* 1994). The experimental group did not differ significantly from the controls in the incidence of preterm delivery (6.7% versus 6.4%) and such interventions as bed rest, hospital admission, or tocolysis (31.6% versus 30.2%). Since the rate of preterm delivery was not modified by routine cervical examinations, it was concluded that either such examinations do not identify women at risk of preterm delivery and/or the interventions prompted by the test are ineffective.

In contrast, several studies in high risk pregnancies have reported that cervical assessment may provide useful information regarding prediction of preterm delivery. In a prospective study of 20 women at high risk for preterm labour, digital vaginal examinations were undertaken at weekly intervals starting from 20-25 weeks and continued until 36 weeks (Catalano *et al* 1989). The state of the cervix was assessed according to the Bishop score and the score added to the prior values in order to obtain a cumulative cervical score. The cumulative score was higher in those that delivered preterm (Figure 1.8).

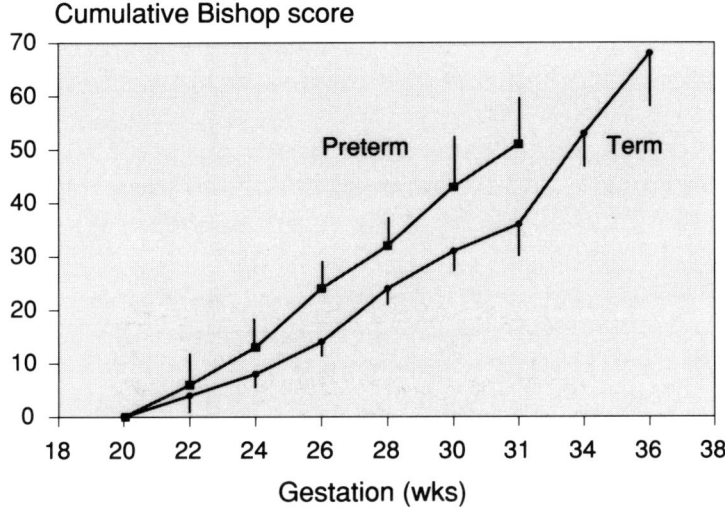

Figure 1.8. Cumulative Bishop score with gestation in patients delivering preterm (■) or at term (●) (mean and standard error; reproduced from Catalano *et al* 1989 with permission).

In another study of 267 women at risk for preterm delivery, a single cervical examination was carried out at 26-28 weeks of gestation and a soft cervix identified 39% of those that subsequently delivered preterm with a false positive rate of 19% (Guinn *et al* 1994).

In two studies, on a total of 301 multiple pregnancies, cervical examinations were performed at one to two weekly intervals from mid-gestation and a score was calculated by subtracting the cervical dilatation from the cervical length in centimetres (Neilson *et al* 1988, Newman *et al* 1991). A score of ≤ 0 at ≤ 34 weeks identified 76% of those that delivered preterm with a false positive rate of 37%.

Recent studies assessing the cervix have used ultrasound examinations. In a study of 201 transvaginal ultrasound examinations at various gestations from booking to term, cervical length was successfully measured in more than 99% of the cases (Sonek *et al* 1990).

Another study compared digital and sonographic assessment of cervical length in women undergoing hysterectomy; ultrasound measurements were very similar to those at pathological examination of the specimens, whereas digital examination provided consistently shorter measurements (Jackson *et al* 1992).

In a transvaginal sonographic study of 177 pregnancies, the length of the cervix was found to decrease linearly with gestation from a mean of 38 mm at 18 weeks to 28 mm at 38 weeks (Figure 1.9); in a group of 32 women who experienced preterm labour, the mean cervical length was significantly lower than those who delivered at term (Murakawa *et al* 1993). Similarly, Andersen *et al* (1990) measured cervical length by transvaginal sonography before 30 weeks of gestation in 113 singleton pregnancies with no risk factors for preterm delivery and reported that, in the group with cervical length below 39 mm, the incidence of subsequent preterm delivery (25%) was significantly higher than in those with a longer cervix (7%).

Cervical assessment by ultrasonography has also been used in women with preterm labour and intact membranes. In two studies on a total of 92 such patients, the cervical length at presentation was less than 30 mm in all 35 patients that delivered preterm and the false positive rate was 47% (Iams *et al* 1994, Murakawa *et al* 1993). Another study of 59 patients in preterm labour demonstrated that ultrasound assessment of cervical length and degree of dilatation of the endocervical canal (funneling) on admission was superior to digital assessment in the prediction of preterm delivery (Gomez *et al* 1994).

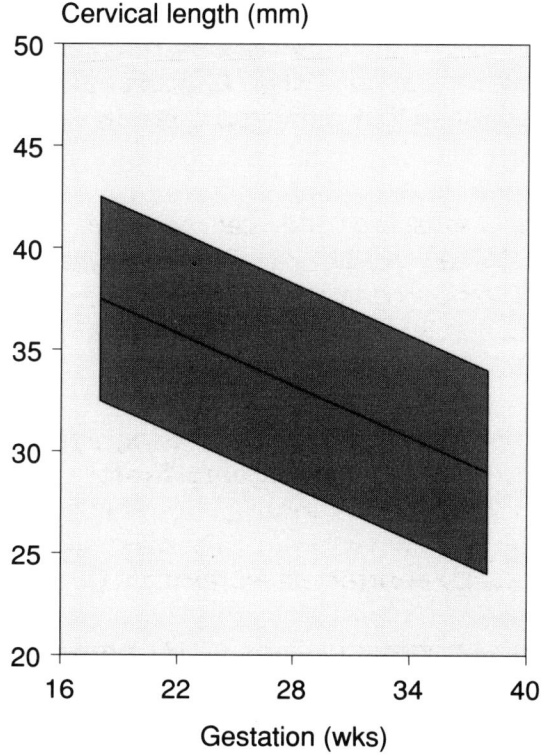

Cervical length (mm)

Gestation (wks)

Figure 1.9. Reference range (mean and standard deviation) of cervical length with gestation, measured by transvaginal sonography (reproduced from Murakawa *et al* 1993 with permission).

PREVENTION OF PRETERM DELIVERY

Intervention on the basis of risk scores

Several studies have used scoring systems to identify high risk pregnancies and investigated the value of antenatal interventions in the prevention of preterm delivery (Table 1.14). Interventions included patient education for the early recognition of the symptoms and signs of preterm labour, increased frequency of clinic visits, psychosocial support and stress reduction classes, dietary advice, and selected prophylactic interventions such as tocolysis, progestogens and bed rest. In some studies the patients were either allocated to intervention or to standard care (Main *et al* 1985, Mueller-Heubach & Guzick 1989, Goldenberg *et al* 1990, Hobel *et al* 1994) and in others the populations examined were compared to historical controls (Herron *et al* 1982, Papiernik *et al* 1985, Meis *et al* 1987b, Yawn and Yawn 1989).

The studies involved a total of 35,246 pregnancies and demonstrated that the antenatal interventions were generally not beneficial in reducing the incidence of preterm delivery.

Table 1.14. Studies that examined the value of intervention programmes based on risk factor scoring.

Author	N	Incidence of preterm delivery	
		Intervention	Controls
Herron *et al* 1982	1,150	4%	7%
Papiernik *et al* 1985	11,356	4%	5%
Main *et al* 1985	132	25%	21%
Meis *et al* 1987b*	17,370	9%	9%
Yawn & Yawn 1989	784	3%	4%
Mueller-Heubach & Guzick 1989	831	22%	21%
Goldenberg *et al* 1990	967	16%	14%
Hobel *et al* 1994	2,654	7%	9%
Total	**35,244**	**8%**	**8%**

* In this study the incidence of birth weight less than 2,500 g was given rather than the incidence of preterm delivery

Intervention on the basis of increased uterine activity

Preterm labour may be preceded by increased uterine activity for several weeks.

Seven randomised studies examined whether home uterine activity monitoring could lead to early detection and prevention of preterm delivery (Table 1.15).

All patients were considered to be at high risk for preterm delivery because of such factors as previous preterm delivery or second trimester loss, vaginal bleeding in the current pregnancy, or multiple pregnancy. One group of patients were managed expectantly with standard care. The other group had home uterine activity monitoring, usually for one hour twice daily, and women with more than three contractions per hour were requested to attend hospital for further assessment and possible tocolytic therapy.

Although some studies found a significantly lower incidence of preterm deliveries in the group that received home monitoring, in the pooled data from all the studies there was no significant difference between the groups in either the incidence of preterm labour or preterm delivery.

Table 1.15. Randomised studies on the value of home uterine activity monitoring in women at high risk of preterm delivery. The study of Knuppel *et al* (1990) was in twin pregnancies and all others in singletons.

Author	N	Preterm labour		Preterm delivery	
		Monitor	**Control**	**Monitor**	**Control**
Morrison *et al* 1987	67	71%	67%	15%	*45%
Iams *et al* 1988	157	-	-	36%	43%
Hill *et al* 1990	245	43%	36%	18%	*43%
Knuppel *et al* 1990	45	74%	62%	50%	*81%
Dyson *et al* 1991	138	34%	34%	13%	6%
Mou *et al* 1991	377	25%	24%	-	-
Blondel *et al* 1992	94	-	-	40%	28%
Total	**1,123**	**38%**	**34%**	**25%**	**29%**

* P < 0.05

Treatment of abnormal cervico-vaginal flora

Two randomised studies, involving a total of 2,252 women with positive genital tract cultures for *Mycoplasma* species at 23-32 weeks of gestation, reported that the incidence of preterm delivery in those that received antibiotics (9%) was not significantly different from the controls (8%; McCormack *et al* 1987, Eschenbach *et al* 1991).

Another prospective study of 142 women with bacterial vaginosis, diagnosed by vaginal swabs taken routinely at 16-27 weeks of gestation, examined the value of treatment with topical clindamycin (2%) cream. Although treatment was associated with microbiologic cure, there was no significant difference in the incidence of preterm delivery between the groups (McGregor *et al* 1994).

Prophylactic use of antibiotics

In a randomised study of 227 pregnancies with no bacteriuria, the administration of tetracycline (250 mg qds) in early pregnancy for six weeks was associated with a significantly lower incidence of preterm delivery (5%) compared to a group that received placebo (15%; Elder *et al* 1971). In another randomised study on 229 pregnancies from a population at high risk for preterm delivery, the patients received either antibiotics (erythromycin 333 mg eight hourly) or placebo for one week at 26-30 weeks of gestation (McGregor *et al* 1990b). There was no significant difference between the groups in either the incidence of preterm delivery or the incidence of preterm prelabour amniorrhexis. Similarly, in a multicentre, randomised study of 938 carriers of *Streptococcus agalactiae*, erythromycin (333 mg 8-hourly) therapy for a period of 10 weeks starting at 28-30 weeks of gestation was not effective at significantly prolonging gestation or reducing the incidence of low birth weight delivery.

Treatment of asymptomatic bacteriuria

The risk for preterm delivery in women with asymptomatic bacteriuria is increased. In eight randomised studies, involving a total of 1,795 women with asymptomatic bacteriuria, antibiotic therapy, compared to placebo, was associated with a significantly lower incidence of preterm delivery (Table 1.16).

Prophylactic use of tocolytics

Randomised studies that examined the value of low-dose β-adrenergic agents in the prevention of preterm labour have demonstrated no benefit in either singleton or twin pregnancies (Table 1.17).

Furthermore, a study of 69 twin pregnancies which had uterine activity monitoring reported that prophylactic tocolytics did not alter the baseline rate of uterine activity or halt the abrupt rise which occurred within 24 hours of labour onset (Garite *et al* 1990).

Table 1.16. Randomised studies of antibiotic therapy for asymptomatic bacteriuria on the incidence of preterm delivery. Some studies reported the incidence of birth weight less than 2,500 g rather than preterm delivery.

Author	N	Incidence of preterm delivery	
		Antibiotics	Controls
Kass 1962	179	7%	*27%
LeBlanc & McGanity 1964	128	7%	*22%
Kincaid-Smith & Bullen 1965	117	15%	21%
Little 1966	265	8%	9%
Savage *et al* 1967	191	8%	*21%
Wren 1969	273	5%	7%
Elder *et al* 1971	229	16%	13%
Brumfitt 1975	413	8%	12%
Total	**1,795**	**9%**	***14%**

* P < 0.05

Table 1.17. Randomised studies on the use of prophylactic tocolysis on the incidence of preterm delivery in singleton (S) and twin (T) pregnancies.

Author	S/T	N	Incidence of preterm delivery	
			Tocolysis	Controls
Briscoe 1966	S	1,165	11%	11%
Mathews *et al* 1967	S	64	6%	6%
Walters & Wood 1977	S	38	14%	6%
Mathews *et al* 1967	T	39	30%	11%
Cetrulo & Freeman 1976	T	84	36%	31%
Marivate *et al* 1977	T	46	30%	30%
O'Conner *et al* 1979	T	48	20%	43%
Skjaerris & Aberg 1982	T	50	28%	40%
Gummerus & Halonen 1987	T	200	37%	37%
Total		**1,734**	**17%**	**17%**

Randomised trials have also assessed the value of progestagens in the prevention of preterm delivery, since one of the hypotheses on the initiation of labour is decrease in progesterone (Csapo *et al* 1971). In a meta-analysis of five studies, on a total of 328 women at high risk of miscarriage or preterm delivery, injections of 17α-hydroxyprogesterone caproate (at least once per week starting during the second or early third trimester of pregnancy) were associated with a significant decrease in the incidence of preterm delivery (16% versus 28% in controls; Keirse 1990). However, there was no significant difference between the groups in the incidence of miscarriage or perinatal death and this therapy has not gained widespread application.

Bed rest

Bed rest is widely prescribed to women whose pregnancies are at higher than average risk of adverse outcome. Early studies in twin pregnancies have suggested that bed rest may be useful in preventing preterm birth (Bender 1952, Persson *et al* 1979). However, in four randomised studies, involving a total of 955 multiple pregnancies, bed rest in hospital or at home from 26 weeks of gestation was not associated with a significant reduction in the incidence of preterm delivery, low birth weight or perinatal death compared to no bed rest (Table 1.18).

Table 1.18. Randomised studies on the effect of bed rest on the incidence of preterm delivery in twin pregnancies.

Author	N	Incidence of preterm delivery	
		Bed rest	**Controls**
Hartikainen-Sorri & Jouppila 1984	154	35%	24%
Saunders *et al* 1985	424	30%	19%
MacLennan *et al* 1990	141	28%	26%
Crowther *et al* 1990	236	62%	67%
Total	**955**	**38%**	**33%**

As with bed rest in twin pregnancies, two randomised studies, involving a total of 351 women with pregnancy-induced hypertension, have found that bed rest was not beneficial in reducing the incidence of preterm delivery or the mean diastolic blood pressure (Matthews 1977, Crowther *et al* 1990).

Cervical cerclage

Cervical cerclage may be effective treatment for cervical incompetence, particularly in women with congenital uterine abnormalities.

A retrospective study of 86 pregnancies with congenital uterine abnormalities, diagnosed by hystero-salpingogram, reported that overall fetal survival was almost twice as high in the group who had been treated with cerclage compared to the untreated group (Seidman *et al* 1991).

Since cervical changes may precede preterm delivery by some weeks, several studies have examined the possible value of prophylactic cerclage in the prevention of preterm delivery. In four randomised studies on a total of 2,042 patients at high risk of mid-trimester losses or preterm delivery, prophylactic cerclage was not associated with a significant decrease in the incidence of preterm delivery either before 37 or 33 weeks (Table 1.19).

Table 1.19. Randomised studies on the effect of prophylactic cervical cerclage on the incidence of preterm delivery. The study of Dor *et al* (1982) was on twin pregnancies and the others on singleton pregnancies.

Author	N	Incidence of preterm delivery	
		Cerclage	Controls
Dor *et al* 1982	50	52%	56%
Lazar *et al* 1984	506	7%	5%
Rush *et al* 1984	194	34%	32%
MRC/RCOG 1993	1,292	26%	31%
Total	**2,042**	**22%**	**25%**

CONCLUSIONS

Preterm birth occurs in less than 10% of deliveries but accounts for more than 60% of neonatal deaths. Survival of preterm infants depends on the gestation at delivery and birth weight, as well as the standard of neonatal care. During the last 30 years the incidence of preterm delivery has not changed but survival of very low birth weight infants has improved dramatically whereas the incidence of disability in survivors has decreased.

Preterm prelabour amniorrhexis complicates about one third of preterm deliveries. The overall survival of preterm infants delivered after prelabour amniorrhexis is no different to those delivered at the same gestation after labour with intact membranes. However, amniorrhexis complicated by intrauterine infection may be associated with a higher perinatal mortality. Similarly, the overall incidence of permanent neurological handicap in infants born prematurely after prelabour amniorrhexis is not higher than in infants born at the same gestation due to other causes. However, infants from pregnancies with intrauterine infection may have developmental delay.

The incidence of postnatal death due to pulmonary hypoplasia in live births decreases from about 50% for those with amniorrhexis before 20 weeks to less than 5% for amniorrhexis after 24 weeks.

The incidence of preterm delivery is highest in teenagers, those that are underweight and those that smoke cigarettes, in women that have had previous preterm deliveries and in women with multiple pregnancy, vaginal bleeding, increased uterine activity, asymptomatic bacteriuria, abnormal vaginal flora, increased cervico-vaginal fibronectin, high vaginal pH and shortening of the cervix.

Attempts at prevention of preterm delivery in high risk pregnancies by such measures as patient education, bed rest, cervical cerclage and prophylactic use of tocolytics or antibiotics have generally been unsuccessful. However, antibiotic therapy for women with asymptomatic bacteriuria is beneficial.

REFERENCES

Alberman E, Botting B. Trends in prevalence and survival of very low birth weight infants, England and Wales; 1983-7. Arch Dis Child 1991;66:1304-9.

Aldous MB, Edmonson MB. Maternal age at first childbirth and risk of low birth weight and preterm delivery in Washington state. JAMA 1993;270:2574-7.

Allen MC, Donohue PK, Dusman AE. The limit of viability-Neonatal outcome of infants born at 22 to 25 weeks gestation. NEJM 1993;329;22:1597-601.

Alvarez H, Caldeyro R. Contractility of the human uterus recorded by new methods. Surg Gynecol Obstet 1950;91:1-13.

Andersen HF, Nugent CE, Wanty SD, Hayashi RH. Prediction of risk for preterm delivery by ultrasonographic measurement of cervical length. Am J Obstet Gynecol 1990;163:859-67.

Bejar R, Wozniak P, Allard M, Benirschke K, Vaucher Y, Coen R, Berry C, Schragg P, Villegas I, Resnick R. Antenatal origin of neurologic damage in newborn infants. Am J Obstet Gynecol 1988;159:357-63.

Bell R. The prediction of preterm labour by recording of spontaneous antenatal uterine activity. Br J Obstet Gynaecol 1983;90:884-7.

Bender S. Twin pregnancy: a review of 472 cases. J Obstet Gynaecol Br Emp 1952;59:510-17.

Beydoun SN, Yasin SY. Premature rupture of the membranes before 28 weeks: Conservative management. Am J Obstet Gynecol 1986;155:471-9.

Blondel B, Breart G, Berthoux Y, Berland M, Mellier G, Rudigoz R, Thoulon J. Home uterine activity monitoring in France: A randomised controlled trial. Am J Obstet Gynecol 1992;167:424-9.

Blott M, Greenough A. Neonatal outcome after prolonged rupture of the membranes starting in the second trimester. Arch Dis Child 1988;63:1146-50.

Briscoe CC. Failure of oral isoxsuprine to prevent prematurity. Am J Obstet Gynecol 1966;95:885-6.

Brumfitt W. The effects of bacteriuria in pregnancy on maternal and fetal health. Kidney Int 1975;8:113-19.

Buekens P, Alexander S, Boutsen M, Blondel B, Kaminski M, Reid M, European Community Collaborative Study Group on Prenatal Screening. Randomised controlled trial of routine cervical examinations in pregnancy. Lancet 1994;344:841-4.

Buttram VC, Gibbons WE. Mullerian anomalies: A proposed classification. Fertil Steril. 1979;32:40-5.

Campbell BA, Newman RB, Stramm SL. Uterine activity after premature rupture of the membranes. Am J Obstet Gynecol 1991;165:422-5.

Carroll R, MacDonald D, Stanley JC. Bacteriuria in pregnancy. Obstet Gynecol 1968;32:525-7.

Carroll SG, Blott M, Nicolaides KH. Preterm prelabour amniorrhexis: Outcome of livebirths. Obstet Gynecol 1995 (In press).

Carver JD, McDermott RJ, Jacobson HN, Sherin KM, Kanarek K, Pimentel B, Tan LH. Infant mortality statistics do not adequately reflect the impact of short gestation. Pediatrics 1993;92:229-32.

Catalano PM, Ashikaga T, Mann LI. Cervical change and uterine activity as predictors of preterm delivery. Am J Perinatol 1989;6:185-9.

Cetrulo CL, Freeman RK. Ritodrine HCL for the prevention of premature labour in twin pregnancies. Acta Genet Med Gemollol 1976;25:321-4.

Cherukuri R, Minkoff H, Feldman J, Parekh A, Glass L. A cohort study of alkaloidal cocaine ("Crack") in pregnancy. Obstet Gynecol 1988;72:147-52.

Collins MH, Moessinger AC, Lleinerman J, James LS, Blanc WA. Morphometry of hypoplastic fetal guinea pig lungs following amniotic fluid leak. Pediatr Res 1986;20:955-60.

Cooke RWI. Trends in preterm survival and incidence of cerebral haemorrhage 1980-9. Arch Dis Child 1991;66:403-7.

Copper RL, Goldenberg RL, Creasy RK, DuBard MB, Davis RO, Enthan SS, Iams JD, Cliver SP. A Multicenter study of preterm birth weight and gestational age specific neonatal mortality. Am J Obstet Gynecol 1993;168:78-84.

Creasy RK, Gummer BA, Liggins GC. System for predicting spontaneous preterm birth. Obstet Gynecol 1980;55:692-5.

Crowther CA, Verkuyl DAA, Bannerman C, Neilson JP, Ashurst HM. The effects of hospitalisation for bed rest on fetal growth, neonatal morbidity, and length of gestation in twin pregnancy. Br J Obstet Gynaecol 1990;97:872-7.

Csapo AI, Knobil E, Van der Molen HJ, Wiest WG. Peripheral plasma progesterone levels during human pregnancy and labour. Am J Obstet Gynecol 1971;110:630-4.

Daikoku NH, Kaltreider DF, Johnson TRB, Johnson JWC, Simmons MA. Premature rupture of membranes and preterm labour: Neonatal infection and perinatal mortality risks. Obstet Gynecol 1981;58:417-25.

Daikoku NH, Kaltreider DF, Khouzami VA, Spence M, Juohnson JWC. Premature rupture of membranes and spontaneous preterm labour: Maternal endometritis risks. Obstet Gynecol 1982;59:13-19.

De Haas I, Harlow BL, Cramer DW, Frigoletto FD. Spontaneous preterm birth: A case control study. Am J Obstet Gynecol 1991;165:1290-6.

Department of Health Statistical Office, Data from Office of Population Census and Surveys. Mortality statistics. Perinatal and infant: Social and biological factors. England and Wales. 1993.

Department of Health Statistics and Research (SR28), Annual summaries of LHS 27/1 returns. United States Annual Vital Statistics Reports. Volume I.Natality. 1989. Department of Health 1993.

Dixon HG, Brant HA. The significance of bacteriuria in pregnancy. Lancet 1967;I:19-20.

Dor J, Shalev J, Mashiach G, Blankstein J, Serr DM. Elective cervical suture of twin pregnancies diagnose ultrasonically in the first trimester following induced ovulation. Gynaecol Obstet Invest 1982;13:55-60.

Dyson DC, Crites YA, Ray DA, Arnstrong MA. Prevention of preterm birth in high risk patients: The role of education and provider contact vs home uterine monitoring. Am J Obstet Gynecol 1991;164:756-62.

Ekwo EE, Gosselink CA, Moawad A. Previous pregnancy outcomes and subsequent risk of preterm rupture of amniotic sac membranes. Br J Obstet Gynaecol 1993;100:536-41.

Ekwo EE, Gosselink CA, Moawad A. Unfavorable outcome in penultimate pregnancy and premature rupture of membranes in succesive pregnancy. Obstet Gynecol 1992;80:166-72.

Elder HA, Santamarina BAG, Smith S, Kass EH. The natural history of asymptomatic bacteriuria during pregnancy: the effect of tetracycline on the clinical course and the outcome of pregnancy. Am J Obstet Gynecol 1971;111:441-57.

Ernest JM, Meis PJ, Moore ML, Swain M. Vaginal pH: A marker of preterm premature rupture of the membranes. Obstet Gynecol 1989;74:734-7.

Eschenbach DA, Nugent RP, Rao AV, Cotch MF, Gibbs RS, Lipscomb KA, Martin DH, Pastorek JG, Rettig PJ, Carey JC, Regan JA, Geromanos KL, Lee MLF, Poole WK, Edelman R, Yaffe SJ, Catz CS, Rhoads GG, McNellis D, et al . A randomised, placebo controlled trial of erythromycin for the treatment of ureoplasma ureolyticum to prevent premature delivery. Am J Obstet Gynecol 1991;164:734-42.

Escobar GJ, Littenberg B, Petitti DB. Outcome among surviving very low birthweight infants: a meta analysis. Arch Dis Child 1991;66:204-11.

Ferrara TB, Hoekstra RE, Couser RJ, Gaziano EP, Calvin SE, Payne NR, Fangman JJ. Survival and follow up of infants born at 23 to 26 weeks of gestational age: Effects of surfactant therapy. J Pediatr 1994;124:119-24.

Ferrara TB, Hoekstra RE, Gaziano E, Knox GE, Couser RJ, Fangman JJ. Changing outcome of extremely premature infants (<26 weeks gestation and <750g): Survival and follow up at a tertiary center. Am J Obstet Gynecol 1989;161:1114-18.

Garite TJ, Bentley DL, Hamer CA, Porto ML. Uterine activity characteristics in multiple gestations. Obstet Gynecol 1990;76:56-9S.

Garite TJ, Freeman RH. Chorioamnionitis in the preterm gestation. Obstet Gynecol 1982;54:539–45.

Gilstrap LC, Leveno KJ, Cunningham FG, Whalley PJ, Roark ML. Renal infection and pregnancy outcome. Am J Obstet Gynecol 1981;141:709-16.

Golan A, Langer R, Bukovsky I, Caspi E. Congenital anomalies of the mullerian system. Fertil Steril 1989;51:747-55.

Golan A, Langer R, Neuman M, Wexler S, Segev E, David MP. Obstetric outcome in women with congenital uterine malformations. J Reprod Med 1992;37:233-7.

Goldenberg RL, Davis RO, Copper RL, Corliss DK, Andrews JB, Carpenter AH. The Alabama Preterm Birth Prevention Project. Obstet Gynecol 1990;75:933-9.

Goldenberg RL, Nelson KG, Dyer RL, Wayne J. The variability of viability: The effect of physicians perceptions of viability on the survival of very low birth weight infants. Am J Obstet Gynecol 1982;143:678-83.

Gomez R, Galasso M, Romero R, Mazor M, Sorokin Y, Goncalves L, Treadwell M. Ultrsonographic examination of the uterine cervix is better than cervical digital examination as a predictor of the likelihood of premature delivery in patients with preterm labour and intact membranes. Am J Obstet Gynecol 1994;171:956-64.

Gower PE, Haswell B, Sidaway ME, DeWardener HE. Follow up of 164 patients with bacteriuria of pregnancy. Lancet 1968;II:990-4.

Gruneberg RN, Leugh DA, Brumfitt W. Relationship of bacteriuria in pregnancy to pyelonephritis, prematurity and fetal mortality. Lancet 1969;II:1-3.

Guinn DA, Wigton TR, Owen J, Socol ML, Frederiksen MC. Prediction of preterm birth in nulliparous patients. Am J Obstet Gynecol 1994;171:1111-15.

Gummerus M, Halonen O. Prophylactic long term oral tocolysis of multiple pregnancies. Br J Obstet Gynaecol 1987;94:249-51.

Gunkel JH et al. Survanta Multidose Study Group. Two yaer follow up of infants treated for neonatal respiratory distress syndrome with bovine surfactant. J Ped. 1994;124:962-7.

Guzick DS, Daikoku NH, Kaltreider DF. Predictability of pregnancy outcome in preterm delivery. Obstet Gynecol 1984;63:645-51.

Hack M, Fanaroff AA. Outcomes of extremely immature infants- a perinatal dilemma. NEJM 1993;329:1649-50.

Hack M, Fanaroff AA. Outcomes of extremely low birth weight infants between 1982 and 1988. NEJM 1989;321:1642-7.

Hack M, Horbar JD, Malloy MH, Tyson JE, Wright E, Wright L. Very low birth weight outcomes of the national institute of child health and human development neonatal network. Pediatrics 1991;87;5:587-96.

Hagen B, Skjeldestad FE. The outcome of pregnancy after CO_2 laser conisation of the cervix. Br J Obstet Gynaecol 1993;100:717-20.

Hardt NS, Kostenbauder M, Ogburn M, Behnke M, Resnick M, Cruz A. Influence of chorioamnionitis on long term prognosis in low birth weight infants. Obstet Gynecol 1985;65:5-9.

Harger JH, Hsing AW, Tuomala RE, Gibbs RS, Mead PB, Eschenbach DA, Knox GE, Polk BF. Risk factors for preterm premature rupture of fetal membranes: A multicenter case control study. Am J Obstet Gynecol 1990;163:130-7.

Hartikainen-Sorri AL, Jouppila P. Is routine hospitalisation needed in the antenatal care of twin pregnancy? J Perinat Med 1984;12:31-4.

Hay PE, Lamont RF, Taylor-Robinson D, Morgan DJ, Ison C, Pearson J. Abnormal bacterial colonisation of the genital tract and subsequent preterm delivery and late miscarriage. BMJ 1994;308:295-8.

Hedegaard M, Henriksen TB, Sabroe S, Secher NJ. Psychological distress in pregnancy and preterm delivery. BMJ 1993;307:234-7.

Heffner LJ, Sherman CB, Speizer FE, Weiss ST. Clinical and environmantal predictors of preterm labour. Obstet Gynecol 1993;81:750-7.

Heinonen K, Hakulinen A, Jokela V. Time trends and determinants of mortality in a very preterm population during the 1980s. Lancet 1988;ii:204-6.

Heinonen PK, Saarikoski S, Pystynen P. Reproductive performance of women with uterine anomalies. Acta Obstet Gynecol Scand 1982;61:157-62.

Herron MA, Katz M, Creasy RK. Evaluation of a preterm birth prevention program: Preliminary report. Obstet Gynecol 1982;59:452-6.

Hill WC, Fleming AD, Martin RW, Hamer C, Knuppel RA, Lake MF, Watson DL, Welch RA, Bentley DL, Gookin KS, Morrison JC. Home uterine activity monitoring is associated with a reduction in preterm birth. Obstet Gynecol 1990;76:13-18S.

Hobel CJ, Ross MG, Bemis RL, Bragonier JR, Nessim S, Sandhu M, Bear MB, Mori B. The West los Angeles Preterm Birth Prevention Project.I. Program impact on high risk women. Am J Obstet Gynecol 1994;170:54-62.

Horbar JD, Wright EC, Onstad L, and Members of the National Institute of Child Health and Human Development Neonatal Research Network. Decreasing mortality associated with the introduction of surfactant therapy: An observational study of neonates weighing between 601 to 1300g at birth. Pediatrics 1993;92;2:191-6.

Howell EM, Vert P. Neonatal intensive care and birth weight specific perinatal mortality in Michigan and Lorraine. Pediatrics 1993;91:464-9.

Iams JD, Johnson FF, Hamer C. Uterine activity and symptoms as predictors of preterm labour. Obstet Gynecol 1990;76:42-6S.

Iams JD, Johnson FF, O'Shaughnessy RW. A prospective randomised trial of home uterine activity monitoring in pregnancies at increased risk of preterm labour. Part II. Am J Obstet Gynecol 1988;159:595-603.

Iams JD, Paraskos J, Landon MB, Teteris JN, Johnson FF. Cervical sonography in preterm labour. Obstet Gynecol 1994;84:40-6.

Jackson GM, Edwin SS, Varner MW, Casal D, Mitchell MD. Regulation of fetal fibronectin production in human chorion cells. Am J Obstet Gynecol 1993;169:1431-5.

Jackson GM, Ludmir J, Bader TJ. The accuracy of digital examination and ultrasound in the evaluation of cervical length. Obstet Gynecol 1992;79:214-18.

Johnson JWC, Daikoku NH, Niebyl JR, Johnson TRB, Khouzami VA, Witter FR. Premature rupture of the membranes and prolonged latency. Obstet Gynecol 1981;57:547-55.

Jones JM, Sweetnam P, Hibbard BM. The outcome of pregnancy after cone biopsy of the cervix: a case control study. Br J Obstet Gynaecol 1979;86:913-16.

Kaltreider DF, Kohl S. Epidemiology of preterm delivery. Clin Obstet Gynecol 1980;23:17-32.

Kari MA, Hallman M, Eronen M, Teramo K, Virtanen M, Koivisto M, Ikonen RS. Prenatal dexamethasone treatment in conjunction with rescue therapy of human surfactant: A randoomised placebo controlled multicenter study. Pediatrics 1994;93:730-6.

Kass EH. Pyelonephritis and bacteriuria. A major problem in preventive medicine. Ann Intern Med 1962;56:46-53.

Katz M, Newman RB, Gill PJ. Assessment of uterine activity in ambulatory patients at high risk of preterm labour and delivery. Am J Obstet Gynecol 1986;154:44-7.

Keirse MJNC. Progestagen administration in pregnancy may prevent preterm delivery. Br J Obstet Gynaecol 1990;97:149-54.

Kilbride HW, Daily DK, Clafin K, Hall RT, Maulik D, Grundy HO. Improved survival and neurodevelopmental outcome for infants less than 801g birthweight. Am J Perinatol 1990;7;2:160-5.

Kincaid-Smith P, Bullen M. Bacteriuria in pregnancy. Lancet 1965;I:395-9.

Kirz DS, Dorchester W, Freeman RK. Advanced maternal age: the mature gravida. Am J Obstet Gynecol 1985;152:7-12.

Kitchen *et al*. The Victorian Infant Collaborative Study Group. Improvement of outcome for infants for birth weight under 1000g. Arch Dis Child 1991;66:765-9.

Klebanoff MA, Shiono PH, Carey JC. The effect of physical activity during pregnancy on preterm delivery and birth weight. Am J Obstet Gynecol 1990;163:1450-6.

Klebanoff MA, Regan JA, Rao V, Nugent RP, Blackwelder WC, Eschenbach DA, Pastorek JG, Williams S, Gibbs RS, Carey JC. Outcome of the Vaginal Infections and Prematurity Study: results of a clinical trial of erythromycin among pregnant women colonized with Group B streptococci. Am J Obstet Gynecol 1995; 172:1540-5

Knuppel RA, Lake MF, Watson DL, Welch RA, Hill WC, Fleming AD, Martin RW, Bentley DL, Moenning RK, Morrison JC. Preventing preterm birth in twin gestation: Home uterine activity monmitoring and perinatal nursing support. Obstet Gynecol 1990;76:24-7S.

Kristensen J, Langhoff-Roos J, Kristensen FB. Increased risk of preterm birth in women with cervical conisation. Obstet Gynecol 1993;81:1005-8.

Kurki T, Ylikorkala O. Coitus during pregnancy is not related to bacterial vaginosis or preterm birth. Am J Obstet Gynecol 1993;169:1130-4.

Layton R. Infection of the urinary tract in pregnancy: an investigation of a new routine in antenatal care. Br J Obstet Gynaecol 1964;71:927-33.

Lazar P, Gueguen S, Dreyfus J, Renaud R, Pontonnier G, Papiernick E. Multicentered controlled trial of cervical cerclage in women at moderate risk of preterm delivery. Br J Obstet Gynaecol 1984;91:731-5.

LeBlanc AL, McGanity WJ. The impact of bacteriuria in pregnancy-a survey of 1300 pregnant patients. Biol Med 1964;22:336-47.

Lehmann DK, Chism J. Pregnancy outcome in medically complicated and uncomplicated patients aged 40 years or older. Am J Obstet Gynecol 1987;157:738-42.

Lieberman E, Lang JM, Ryan KJ, Monson RR, Schoenbaum SC. The association of inter pregnancy interval with small for gestational age births. Obstet Gynecol 1989;74:1-5.

Lieberman E, Ryan KJ, Monson RR, Schoenbaum SC. Risk factors accounting for racial differences in the rate of premature birth. NEJM 1987;317:743-8.

Linn S, Schoenbaum SC, Monson RR, Rosner B, Stubblefield PG, Ryan KJ. The relationship between induced abortion and outcome of subsequent pregnancies. Am J Obstet Gynecol 1983;146:136-40.

Little PJ. The incidence of urinary infection in 5000 pregnant women. Lancet 1966;II:925-8.

Lockwood CJ, Senyei AE, Dische MR, Casal D, Shah KD, Thung SN, Jones L, Deligdische L, Garite TJ. Fetal fibronectin in cervical and vaginal secretions as a predictor of preterm delivery. NEJM 1991;325:669-74.

Lockwood CJ, Wein R, Lapinski R, Casal D, Berkowitz G, Alvarez M, Berkowitz RL. The presence of cervical and vaginal fetal fibronectin predicts delivery in an inner city obstetric population. Am J Obstet Gynecol 1993;169:798-804.

Lucas A, Morley R, Cole TJ, Bamford MF, Boon A, Crowle P, Dossetor JFB, Pearse R. Maternal fatness and viability of preterm infants. BMJ 1988;296:1495-7.

Lyon AJ, Clarkson P, Jeffrey I, West GA. Effect of ethnic origin of the mother on fetal outcome. Arch Dis Child 1994;70:F40-3.

MacLennan AH, Green RC, O'Shea R, Brookes C, Morris D. Routine hospital admission in twin pregnancy between 26 and 30 weeks' gestation. Lancet 1990;335:267-9.

Madinger NE, Greenspoon JS, Ellrodt AG. Pneumonia during pregnancy: has modern technology improved maternal and fetal outcome? Am J Obstet Gynecol 1989;161:657-62.

Main DM, Gabbe SG, Richardson D, Strong S. Can preterm deliveries be prevented? Am J Obstet Gynecol 1985;151:892-8.

Major CA, Kitzmiller JL. Perinatal survival with expectant management of midtrimester rupture of membranes. Am J Obstet Gynecol 1990;163:838-44.

Marivate M, De Villiers KQ, Fairbrother P. Effect of prophylactic outpatient administration of fenoterol on the time and onset of spontaneous labour and fetal growth rate in twin pregnancy. Am J Obstet Gynecol 1977;128:707-8.

Martin JN, McColgin SW, Martin RW, Roach H, Morrison JC. Uterine activity among a diverse group of patients at high risk of preterm delivery. Obstet Gynecol 1990;76:47-50S.

Martin RW, Gookin KS, Hill WC, Fleming AD, Knuppel RA, Lake MF, Watson DL, Welch RA, Bently DL, Morrison JC. Uterine activity compared with symptomatology in the detection of preterm labour. Obstet Gynecol 1990;76:19-22S.

Mathews DD. A randomised controlled trial of bed rest and sedation or normal activity and non sedation in the management of non-albuminuric hypertension in late pregnancy. Br J Obstet Gynaecol 1977;84:108-14.
Mathews DD, Friend JB, Michael CA. A double blind trial of oral isoxuprine in the prevention of premature labour. J Obstet Gynaecol Br Commnwlth 1967;74:68-70.

McCormack WM, Rosner B, Lee Y, Munoz A, Charles D, Kass EH. Effect on birthweight of erythromycin traetment of pregnant women. Obstet Gynecol 1987;69:202-7.

McGregor JA, French JI, Jones W, Milligan K, McKinney PJ, Patterson E, Parker R. Bacterial vaginosis is associated with prematurity and vaginal fluid mucinase and sialidase: Results of a controlled trial of topical clindamycin cream. Am J Obstet Gynecol 1994;170:1048-60.

McGregor JA, French JI, Richter R, Franco-Buff A, Johnson A, Hillier S, Judson FN, Todd JK. Antenatal microbiologic and maternal risk factors associated with prematurity. Am J Obstet Gynecol 1990a;163:1465-73.

McGregor JA, French JI, Richter R, Vuchetich M, Bachus V, Seo K, Hillier S, Judson FN, McFee J, Schoonmaker J, Todd JK. Cervicovaginal microflora and pregnancy outcome: Results of a double blind, placebo controlled trial of erythromycin treatment. Am J Obstet Gynecol 1990b;163:1580-91.

McGregor SN, Keith LG, Chasnoff IJ, Rosner MA, Chisum GM, Shaw P, Minogue JP. Cocaine use dueing pregnancy: Adverse perinatal outcome. Am J Obstet Gynecol 1987;157:686-90.

McKenzie H, Donnet ML, Howie PW, Patel NB, Benvie DT. Risk of preterm delivery in pregnant women with group B streptococcal urinary infections or urinary antibodies to group B streptococcal and E.coli antigens. Br J Obstet Gynaecol 1994;101:107-13.

Meis PJ, Ernest JM, Moore ML. Causes of low birth weight births in public and private patients. Am J Obstet Gynecol 1987a;156:1165-8.

Meis PJ, Ernest JM, Moore ML, Michielutte R, Sharp PC, Buescher PA. Regional program for prevention of premature birth in northwestern North Carolina. Am J Obstet Gynecol 1987b;157:550-6.

Michalas SP. Outcome of pregnancy in women with uterine malformation:evaluation of 62 cases. Int J Gynecol Obstet 1991;35:215-19.

Mitchell MC, Lerner E. Weight gain and pregnancy outcome in underweight and normal weight women. J Am J Obstet Gynecol Diet Assoc 1989;641:634-8.

Moessinger AC, Collins MH, Blanc WA, Rey HR, James LS. Oligohydramnios-induced lung hypoplasia: the influence of timing and duration and gestation. Pediatr Res 1986;20:951-4.

Monga M, Chmieloweic S, Andres RL, Troyer LR, Parisi VM. Cocaine alters placental production of thromboxane and prostacyclin. Am J Obstet Gynecol 1994;171:965-9.

Morales WJ. Talley T. Premature rupture of membranes at <25 weeks: A management dilemma. Am J Obstet Gynecol 1993;168:503-7.

Morales WJ. The effect of chorioamnionitis on the developmental outcome of preterm infants at one year. Obstet Gynecol 1987;70:183-6.

Moretti M, Sibai BM. Maternal and perinatal outcome of expectant management of premature rupture of membranes in the midtrimester. Am J Obstet Gynecol 1988;159:390-6.

Morrison JC, Martin JN, Martin RW, Gookin KS, Wiser WL. Prevention of preterm birth by ambulatory assessement of uterine activity: A randomised study. Am J Obstet Gynecol 1987;156:536-43.

Morrison JC, Martin RW, Johnson C, Hess LW. Characteristics of uterine activity in gestations less than 20 weeks. Obstet Gynecol 1990;76:60-3S.

Mou SM, Sunderji SG, Gall S, How H, Patel V, Gray M, Kayne HL, Corwin M. Mulicenter randomised clinical trial of home uterine activity monitoring for detection of preterm labour. Am J Obstet Gynecol 1991;165:858-66.

MRC/RCOG Working Party on Cervical Cerclage. Final report of the Medical research Council/Royal College of Obstetricians and Gynaecologists Multicentre Randomised Trial of Cervical Cerclage. Br J Obstet Gynaecol 1993;100:516-23.

Mueller-Heubach E, Guzick DS. Evaluation of risk scoring in a preterm birth prevention study of indigent patients. Am J Obstet Gynecol 1989;160:829-37.

Murakawa H, Utumi T, Hasegawa I, Tanaka K, Fuzimori R. Evaluation of threatened preterm delivery by transcervical ultrasonographic measurement of cervical length. Obstet Gynecol 1993;82:829-32.

Murphy JF, Dauncey M, Newcombe R. Employment in pregnancy:prevalence, maternal characteristics, perinatal outcome. Lancet 1984;I:1163-6.

Naeye RL & Peters EC. Causes and consequences of premature rupture of fetal membranes. Lancet 1980;I:192-4.

Nageotte MP, Casal D, Senyei. Fetal fibronectin in patients at increased risk for premature birth. Am J Obstet Gynecol 1994;170:20-5.

Nageotte MP, Dorchester W, Porto M, Keegan KA, Freeman RK. Quantitation of uterine activity preceding preterm, term and postterm labour. Am J Obstet Gynecol 1988;158:1254-9.

Nandi C, Nelson MR. Maternal pregravid weight, age, and smoking status as risk factors for low birth weight births. Pub Health Rep 1992;107:658-61.

Narahara H, Johnston JM. Smoking and preterm labour: Effect of cigarette smoke extract on the secretion of platelet activating factor acetylhydrolase by human decidual macrophages. Am J Obstet Gynecol 1993;169:1321-6.

Neilson JP, Mutambira M. Coitus, twin pregnancy, and preterm labour. Am J Obstet Gynecol 1989;160:416-18.

Neilson JP, Verkuyl DAA, Crowther CA, Bannerman C. Preterm labour in twin pregnancies: Prediction by cervical assessement. Obstet Gynecol 1988;72:719-23.

Newman RB, Godsey RK, Ellings JM, campbell BA, Eller DP, Miller MC. Quantification of cervical change: relationship to preterm delivery in the multifetal gestation. Am J Obstet Gynecol 1991;165:264-71.

Newman RB, Richmond GS, Winston YE, Hamer C, Katz M. Antepartum uterine activity characteristics differentiating true from threatened preterm labour. Obstet Gynecol 1990;76:39-41S.

Nimrod C, Varela-Gittings F, Machin G, Campbell D, Wesenberg R. The effect of very prolonged membrane rupture on fetal development. Am J Obstet Gynecol 1984;148:540-3.

O'Conner MC, Murphy H, Dalrymple IJ. Double blind trial of ritodrine and placebo in twin pregnancy. Br J Obstet Gynaecol 1979;86:706-9.

Office of Population Census and Surveys. Mortality statistics. Perinatal and infant: Social and biological factors.England and Wales. 1991.

Owen J, Baker SL, Hauth JC, Goldenberg RL, Davis RO, Copper RL. Is indicated or spontaneous preterm delivery more advantageous for the fetus? Am J Obstet Gynecol 1990a;163:868-72.

Owen J, Goldenberg RL, Davi RO, Kirk KA, Copper RL. Evaluation of a risk scoring system as a predictor of preterm birth in an indigent population. Am J Obstet Gynecol 1990b;163:873-9.

Papiernik E, Bouyer J, Dreyfus J, Collin D, Winisdorffer G, Guegen S, Lecomte M, Lazar P. Prevention of preterm births: A perinatal study in Haguenau, France. Pediatrics 1985;76:154-8.

Patrick MJ. Influence of maternal renal infection on the fatus and infant. Arch Dis Child 1967;42:208-13.

Persson PH, Grennert L, Gennser G, Kullander S. An improved outcome in twin pregnancies. Acta Obstet Gynecol Scand 1979;58:3-7.

Phelps DL, Brown DR, Tung B, Cassady G, McClead RE, Purohit DM, Palmer EA. 28 day survival rates of 6676 neonates with birth weights of 1250 grams or less. Pediatrics 1991;87:7-17.

Powers W, Hegwood PD. Survival and ventilatory course of a regional cohort of very low birthweight (501-1500g) infants. Am J Perinatol 1989;6;4:427-31.

Resnick MB, Carter RL, Ariet M, Bucciarelli RL, Evans JH, Furlough RR, Ausbon WW, Curran JS. Effect of birth weight, race, and sex on survival of low birth weight infants in neonatal intensive care. Am J Obstet Gynecol 1989;161:184-7.

Riedewald S, Kreutzmann I, Heinze T, Saling E. Vaginal and cervical pH in normal pregnancy and pregnancy comlicate by preterm labour. J Perinat Med 1990;18:181-5.

Robertson JG, Livingstone JRB, Isdale MH. The management and complications of asymptomatic bacteriuria in pregnancy. Br J Obstet Gynaecol 1968;75:59-65.

Robichaux AG, Stedman CM, Hamer C. Uterine activity in patients with cervical cerclage. Obstet Gynecol 1990;76:63-6S.

Rotschild A, Ling EW, Puterman ML, Farquharson D. Neonatal outcome after prolonged preterm rupture of the membranes. Am J Obstet Gynecol 1990;162:46-52.

Rush RW, Davey DA, Segall ML. The effect of preterm delivery on perinatal mortality. Br J Obstet Gynaecol 1978;85:806-11.

Rush RW, Isaacs S, McPherson K, Jones L, Chalmers I, Grant A. A randomised controlled trial of cervical cerclage in women at high risk of preterm delivery. Br J Obstet Gynaecol 1984;91:724-30.

Rush RW, Keirse MJNC, Howat P, Baum JD, Anderson ABM, Turnbull AC. Contribution of preterm delivery to perinatal mortality. BMJ 1976;2:965-8.

Sanjose S, Roman E, Beral V. Low birthweight and preterm delivery, Scotland,1981-84: effect of parents occupation. Lancet 1991;338:428-30.

Saunders MC, Dick JS, Brown I, McPherson K, Chalmers I. The effects of hospital admission for bed rest on the duration of twin pregnancy. A randomised trial. Lancet 1985;II:793-5.

Savage WE, Hajj SN, Kass EH. Demograohic and prognostic characteristics of bacteriuria in pregnancy. Medicine 1967;46:385-407.

Schreiber J, Benedetti T. Conservative management of preterm premature rupture of the fetal membranes in a low socio-economic population. Am J Obstet Gynecol 1980;136:92-6.

Seidman DS, Ben-Rafael Z, Bider D, Recabi K, Mashiach S. the role of cervical cerclage in the management of uterine anomalies. Surg Gynecol Obstet 1991;173:384-6.

Shennan AT, Milligan JE, Hoskins EM. Perinatal factors associated with death or handicap in very preterm infants. Am J Obstet Gynecol. 1985:151:231-8.

Skjaerris J, Aberg A. Prevention of prematurity in twin pegnancies by orally administered terbutaline. Acta Obstet Gynecol Scand 1982;108:39-40.

Sonek JD, Iams JD, Blumenfeld M, Johnson F, Landon M, Gabbe S. Measurement of cervical length in pregnancy: Comparison between vaginal ultrsonography and digital examination. Obstet Gynecol 1990;76:172-6.

Spence MR, Williams R, DiGregorio GJ, Kirby-McDonnell A, Polansky M. The relationship between recent cocaine use and pregnancy outcome. Obstet Gynecol 1991;78:326.

Taylor J, Garite TJ. Premature rupture of membranes before fetal viability. Obstet Gynecol 1984;64:615-20.

Thompson P, Greenough A, Nicolaides KH, Blott M. Chronic respiratory morbidity following prolonged and preterm rupture of membranes. Arch Dis Child 1990;65:878-80.

Toth M, Witkin SS, Ledger W, Thaler H. The role of infection in the aetiology of preterm birth. Obstet Gynecol 1988;71:723-6.

Tucker JM, Goldenberg RL, Davis RO, Copper RL, Winkler CL, Hauth JC. Etiologies of preterm birth in an indigent population: Is prevention a logical expectation? Obstet Gynecol 1991;77:343-7.

Van Reempts P, Kegelaers B, Van Dam K, Van Overmeire. Neonatal outcome after very prolonged and premature rupture of membranes. Am J Perinatol 1993;10;4:288-91.

Varner MW, Galsk RP. Conservative management of premature rupture of the membranes. Am J Obstet Gynecol 1981;140:39-43.

Vermont-Oxford Trials Network Database Project. The Vermont-Oxford trials Network: Very low birth weight outcomes for 1990. Pediatrics 1993;91:540-5.

Victorian Infant Collaborative Study Group. Improvement of outcome for infants for birth weight under 1000g. Arch Dis Child 1991;66:765-9.

Virji SK, Cottington E. Risk factors associated with preterm deliveries among racial groups in a national sample of married mothers. Am J Perinatol 1991;8:347-50.

Walters WAW, Wood C. A trial of oral ritodrine for the prevention of premature labour. Br J Obstet Gynaecol 1977;84:26-30.

Wen SW, Goldengerg RL, Cutter GR, Hoffman HJ, Cliver SP. Intrauterine growth retardation and preterm delivery: prenatal risk factors in an indigent population. Am J Obstet Gynecol 1990;162:213-18.

Whyte HE, Fitzhardinge PM, Shennan AT, Lennox K, Smith L, Lacy J. Extreme immaturity: Outcome of 568 pregnancies of 23-26 weeks gestation. Obstet Gynecol 1993;82:1-7.

Wolf EJ, Vintzileos AM, Rosenkrantz TS, Rodis JF, Salafia CM, Pezzullo JG. Do survival and morbidity of very low birth weight infants vary according to the primary pregnancy complication that results in preterm delivery? Am J Obstet Gynecol 1993;169:1233-9.

Wood B, Katz V, Bose C, Goolsby R, Kraybill E. Survival and morbidity of extremely premature infants based on obstetric assessment of gestational age. Obstet Gynecol 1989;74:889-92.

Working Group on the Very Low Birthweight Infant. European Community collaborative study of outcome of pregnancy between 22 and 28 weeks gestation. Lancet 1990;336:782-4.

Wren BG. Subclinical renal infection and prematurity. Med J Aust 1969;II:596-600.

Yawn BP & Yawn RA. Preterm birth prevention in a rural practice. JAMA 1989;262:230-3.

Zuckerman B, Frank DA, Hingson R, Amaro H, Levensen SM, Kayne H, Parker S, Vinci R, Aboage K, Fried LE, Cabral H, Timperi R, Bauchner H. Effects of maternal marijuana and cocaine use on fetal growth. NEJM 1989;320:762-8.

Zuckerman BS, Walker DK, Frank DA, Chase C, Hamburg B. Adolescent pregnancy: Biobehavioural determinants of outcome. J Pediatr 1984;105:857-62.

Infection: amniorrhexis, preterm delivery, neonatal sepsis

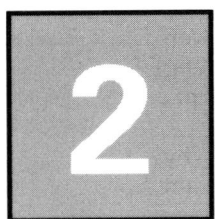

OVERVIEW

INFECTION AS A CAUSE OF AMNIORRHEXIS
    Incidence of positive amniotic fluid cultures
    The lower genital tract as the source of infection
    Membrane structure and amniorrhexis
    Infection as cause rather than consequence of amniorrhexis
    Host defence against infection

INFECTION AS A CAUSE OF PRETERM DELIVERY
    Interval from amniorrhexis to delivery
    Intrauterine infection, cytokines and prostaglandins

INTRAUTERINE INFECTION AND RISK OF NEONATAL SEPSIS
    Diagnosis of neonatal sepsis
    Incidence of neonatal sepsis
    Mortality from neonatal sepsis

CONCLUSION

OVERVIEW

In a high proportion of pregnancies complicated by preterm labour and preterm prelabour amniorrhexis, the underlying cause may be ascending infection from the lower genital tract. Thus, positive amniotic fluid cultures, with organisms commonly found in the vagina, are present in about one tenth of pregnancies in preterm labour with intact membranes and in more than one third of cases with preterm prelabour amniorrhexis. Additionally, in-vitro studies have demonstrated that, although micro-organisms can cross intact chorioamniotic membranes, they can also cause damage to membranes by the release of various proteases and this damage is augmented by the host response to infection.

In preterm prelabour amniorrhexis, the evidence that infection may be the cause of subsequent preterm labour and delivery is based on the demonstration that in the group with intrauterine infection (i) spontaneous delivery occurs earlier than in those without infection, and (ii) there is increased amniotic fluid concentration of prostaglandins, leukotrienes and a variety of inflammatory mediators, that can induce uterine contractions. Animal studies have shown that intra-amniotic inoculation of bacteria causes labour which is preceded by an increase in the amniotic fluid concentration of first cytokines and then prostaglandins.

The consequences of intrauterine infection are preterm delivery and neonatal sepsis. The incidence of neonatal sepsis in the general population is about 0.4%, but the incidence in patients with preterm prelabour amniorrhexis and positive amniotic fluid cultures is 20 times higher.

INFECTION AS A CAUSE OF AMNIORRHEXIS

Incidence of positive amniotic fluid cultures

Studies of amniotic fluid obtained by amniocentesis during preterm labour with intact membranes have reported positive cultures in about one tenth of the pregnancies (Table 2.1), whereas, in preterm prelabour amniorrhexis, about one third of pregnancies had positive cultures (Table 2.2). In those studies that also tested for *Mycoplasma* species, the incidence of infection was even higher.

Table 2.1. Incidence of positive amniotic fluid cultures in pregnancies with preterm labour and intact membranes. The mean incidence of positive cultures in those studies that cultured the fluid only for aerobic and anaerobic organisms was 9%, whereas in those that also examined for *Mycoplasma* species the incidence was 14% (*).

Author	Gestation	N	Positive cultures
Wahbeh *et al* 1984	<35 wks	33	21%
Gravett *et al* 1986	<35 wks	54	24%*
Leigh & Garite 1986	<37 wks	59	11%
Skoll *et al* 1989	<36 wks	127	5%*
Dunlow & Duff 1990	<37 wks	72	1%
O'Brien *et al* 1990	<36 wks	50	10%
Gauthier *et al* 1991	<34 wks	113	16%*
Romero *et al* 1991	<37 wks	195	12%*
Coultrip & Grossman 1992	<35 wks	107	11%*
Watts *et al* 1992	<35 wks	105	19%*
Hillier *et al* 1993	<34 wks	50	18%*
Total		**214/751***	**9%/14%***

Table 2.2. Incidence of positive amniotic fluid cultures in pregnancies with preterm prelabour amniorrhexis. The mean incidence of positive cultures in those studies that cultured the fluid only for aerobic and anaerobic organisms was 24%, whereas in those that also examined for *Mycoplasma* species the incidence was 36% (*).

Author	Gestation	N	Positive cultures
Garite & Freeman 1982	<35 wks	86	23%
Cotton *et al* 1984	<37 wks	41	14%
Broekhuizen *et al* 1985	<37 wks	53	28%
Vintzileos *et al* 1986	<35 wks	54	22%
Fisk *et al* 1987	<34 wks	20	30%
Romero *et al* 1988a	<37 wks	221	29%*
O'Brien *et al* 1990	<36 wks	27	37%
Dudley *et al* 1991	<37 wks	79	37%*
Coultrip & Grossman 1992	<37 wks	29	41%*
Gauthier *et al* 1992	<35 wks	111	48%*
Carroll *et al* 1995a	<37 wks	82	36%*
Total		**281/522***	**24%/36%***

Although in preterm prelabour amniorrhexis the incidence of positive amniotic fluid cultures is about 40% (Table 2.2), the incidence of histological chorioamnionitis (see Chapter 3) is about 50% (Table 2.3) and is inversely related to the gestation at amniorrhexis (Hillier *et al* 1988, Kitajima *et al* 1992). These findings suggest that amniotic fluid cultures may underestimate the contribution of infection to preterm prelabour amniorrhexis. Alternatively, histological chorioamnionitis does not necessarily imply infection; in about one third of cases of histological chorioamnionitis, placental cultures are negative (see Chapter 3).

Table 2.3. Incidence of histological chorioamnionitis in preterm prelabour amniorrhexis.

Author	Amniorrhexis	N	Chorioamnionitis
Kappy *et al* 1979	<37 wks	110	29%
Ismail *et al* 1985	<37 wks	100	63%
Guzick & Winn 1985	<37 wks	105	47%
Fisk *et al* 1987	<37 wks	51	59%
Zlatnik *et al* 1990	<35 wks	27	56%
Mueller-Heubach *et al* 1990	<37 wks	88	42%
Total		**481**	**47%**

The lower genital tract as the source of infection

Animal studies

Animal models support the hypothesis that organisms from the cervix can enter the amniotic cavity and cause intra-amniotic infection and pregnancy loss.

In a study involving 80 pregnant rabbits, endocervical inoculation of *E. coli* was associated with a significant increase (compared to a control group that had received only saline) in the incidence of fever, vaginal bleeding and pregnancy loss (Heddleston *et al* 1993). At the end of the experiment all animals were sacrificed and at postmortem examination the incidence of positive decidual or amniotic fluid cultures was 97%, compared to 0% for the controls. Furthermore, treatment with antibiotics from the time of inoculation was associated with reduced incidence of positive cultures and symptoms of infection (Heddleston *et al* 1993).

Studies in twins

In a study of 46 twin pregnancies in preterm labour with intact membranes, amniotic fluid was obtained from both sacs by amniocentesis (Romero *et al* 1990). A positive amniotic fluid culture in at least one sac was noted in 11% of patients and in all cases the presenting sac was involved, with or without infection of the second sac. Furthermore, in the majority of cases, the same organism was found in both sacs and the inoculum size was always larger in the presenting one.

Types of organisms

In patients with preterm prelabour amniorrhexis and positive amniotic fluid cultures, a wide range of organisms has been isolated and the most frequent were *Mycoplasma* species, *Streptococcus agalactiae*, *Bacteroides* and *Gardnerella vaginalis* (Table 2.4). These organisms are the ones commonly found in the vagina.

Table 2.4. Prevalence of organisms isolated from amniotic fluid obtained by amniocentesis from a total of 618 pregnancies with preterm prelabour amniorrhexis (Garite & Freeman 1982, Cotton *et al* 1984, Broekhuizen *et al* 1985, Vintzileos *et al* 1986, Romero *et al* 1988a, Coultrip & Grossman 1992, Gauthier *et al* 1992, Carroll *et al* 1995a).

Organism	Prevalence	Organism	Prevalence
Mycoplasma species	20.9%	*Candida albicans*	0.8%
Streptococcus	3.5%	*Haemophilus influenzae*	0.8%
Streptococcus viridans	1.3%	Diphtheroids	0.5%
Peptostreptococcus	2.3%	*Klebsiella*	0.5%
Streptococcus other	3.4%	*Citrobacter*	0.2%
Bacteroides	3.4%	*Clostridia*	0.2%
Gardnerella vaginalis	3.4%	*Cryseomonas*	0.2%
Escherichia coli	1.6%	*Enterobacter*	0.2%
Fusobacterium	1.6%	*Proteus*	0.2%
Neisseria gonorrhoeae	1.1%	*Pseudomonas*	0.2%

In one of the studies involving 97 cases of preterm prelabour amniorrhexis, cultures of cervico-vaginal swabs and amniotic fluid demonstrated that, in about 75% of the cases with positive amniotic fluid cultures, the same organisms were isolated from the lower genital tract (Carroll *et al* 1995a; see Chapter 3).

As with amniotic fluid cultures (Table 2.4), studies which have examined placental cultures have also reported that the organisms recovered are similar to those commonly found in the vagina (Table 2.5).

Table 2.5. Prevalence of organisms isolated from placental cultures (Pankuch *et al* 1984, Svensson *et al* 1986, Quinn *et al* 1987, Hillier *et al* 1988, Zlatnick *et al* 1990).

Organism	N	Prevalence
Streptococcus viridans	357	6%
Streptococcus agalactiae	245	5%
Peptostreptococcus	293	12%
Bacteroides	357	4%
Gardnerella vaginalis	207	7%
Mycoplasma species	250	30%

Further evidence implicating the lower genital tract as the source of infection is derived from studies of women with bacterial vaginosis. This condition is characterised by depletion of Lactobacilli with greatly increased numbers of *Gardnerella vaginalis* in association with such organisms as *Bacteroides*, *Peptostreptococci* and *Mycoplasma* species. Bacterial vaginosis, found in 10-15% of pregnant women (Hay *et al* 1994) is associated with increased risk of preterm delivery and preterm prelabour amniorrhexis (McDonald *et al* 1991, Kurki *et al* 1992, McGregor *et al* 1993, Hay *et al* 1994). Furthermore, in patients with bacterial vaginosis that develop intra-amniotic infection, the pattern of organisms found in amniotic fluid is the same as that found in the vagina (Silver *et al* 1989).

Membrane structure and amniorrhexis

The fetal membranes are a complex structural and metabolic tissue which play a central role in the maintenance of the intrauterine environment and are involved in many of the physiological processes of labour and delivery.

The membranes consist of multiple layers, comprising amniotic epithelium and basement membrane, connective tissue, chorion and decidua (Malak & Bell 1994). The connective tissue is composed mainly of collagen types I and III which provide the tensile strength of the membranes (Klima & Schmidt 1988, Klima *et al* 1989). The arrangement of collagen fibres is such that there are randomly distributed 'weak spots' at increased risk for amniorrhexis (Schmidt & Klima 1989).

In-vitro studies have demonstrated that towards term the membranes become thinner due to cell destruction by apoptosis, and the collagen concentration decreases (Skinner *et al* 1981, Easterling *et al* 1993). There is a concomitant decrease in the tensile strength of membranes with gestation (Lavery and Miller 1979).

Light microscopic studies of membranes obtained after spontaneous delivery at term have demonstrated a focal area of structural weakness from which amniorrhexis starts; subsequently the tear is extended to involve the adjacent areas (Malak & Bell 1994).

Preterm amniorrhexis

There is contradictory evidence as to whether the total collagen content of membranes that rupture prematurely is reduced (Skinner *et al* 1981) or normal (Evaldson *et al* 1987). However, the membranes from pregnancies with preterm amniorrhexis have increased collagenolytic activity, higher collagen solubility and lower collagen synthesis (Vadillo-Ortega *et al* 1990), especially of type III collagen (Kanayama *et al* 1985).

Bacteria-induced amniorrhexis

A study of placental histology, after delivery at 18-40 weeks of gestation, reported that with advancing gestation there is disappearance of the trophoblast layer and membrane thinning; this process was accelerated in cases with evidence of histological chorioamnionitis (Parmley 1990). Micro-organisms present in the lower genital tract produce a variety of proteases which can damage the membranes directly (McGregor *et al* 1986, McGregor *et al* 1987). Infection-mediated amniorrhexis may also be due to activation of fibroblasts and consequent increase in collagenase activity (Vadillo-Ortega *et al* 1991). Additionally, micro-organisms may produce chemotactic factors to induce a host response which itself causes membrane damage (McGregor *et al* 1986). In-vitro studies, involving culture of common genital tract organisms in vessels containing chorioamniotic membrane preparations, have reported that bacteria can cause mechanical weakening of the membranes which is enhanced by the presence of neutrophils (Sbarra *et al* 1987, Schoonmaker *et al* 1989).

Membrane permeability to leukocytes and bacteria

Electron microscopic studies have demonstrated that the amnion is not a mechanical barrier to cells of the inflammatory system; polymorphonuclear leukocytes can easily migrate through intact membranes by adhesion to basement membrane and subsequent local partial proteolysis of the matrix and active movement through the loose stroma (Bakowski & Tschesche 1992). Such studies have also demonstrated that certain bacteria, such as *E. coli* and group B streptococci, have the ability to cross intact membranes (Galask *et al* 1984, Gyr *et al* 1994).

Infection as cause rather than consequence of amniorrhexis

If the amniotic membranes protected against ascending organisms, the incidence of intrauterine infection would be expected to increase with time after amniorrhexis. In contrast, if one of the causes of amniorrhexis was infection, then the incidence of chorioamnionitis would decrease with time after amniorrhexis.

In three series with a total of 242 patients with preterm prelabour amniorrhexis at 16-27 weeks of gestation, the pregnancies were managed expectantly (Taylor & Garite 1984, Moretti & Sibai 1988, Major & Kitzmiller 1990). Clinical chorioamnionitis was diagnosed in 54% of the patients that delivered within three days of amniorrhexis; subsequently, the incidence of chorioamnionitis did not change with the interval from amniorrhexis and remained at about 30%.

The findings of these studies suggest that in some cases infection may be the cause of amniorrhexis (those cases that develop clinical signs within a few days of amniorrhexis). However, the findings are also compatible with the hypothesis that amniorrhexis may predispose to intrauterine infection since a high proportion of patients, that were originally well, developed clinical chorio-amnionitis several days or weeks after amniorrhexis. Another explanation for these findings is that clinical signs of chorioamnionitis do not constitute sensitive and specific markers of intrauterine infection and, as shown in Chapter 3, this may well be the case.

In a study of 69 pregnancies with preterm prelabour amniorrhexis at 12-36 weeks of gestation, the diagnosis of intrauterine infection was based on the results of culture of amniotic fluid and fetal blood obtained by amniocentesis and cordocentesis, respectively (Carroll *et al* 1995b). In patients with fetal bacteraemia, there was spontaneous delivery within five days of amniorrhexis, whereas in those with negative fetal blood and amniotic fluid cultures the interval between amniorrhexis and delivery was prolonged by up to five months and subsequent cultures of blood obtained from the umbilical cord at delivery or from the neonates were negative. These findings are compatible with the hypothesis that infection is the cause rather than the consequence of amniorrhexis.

Host defence against infection

Cervical mucus

Cervical mucus provides an interface between the environments of the vagina, the endocervix and fetal membranes and is composed of a non-newtonian hydrogel with large meshes of up to 5 microns in size (Volochine *et al* 1988). In addition to its possible action as a mechanical barrier to microorganisms, cervical mucus has intrinsic antibacterial activity. It contains non-specific antibacterial agents, such as lactoferrin and lysozyme. The concentration of these factors is lower in patients with preterm labour and chorioamnionitis compared to those in preterm labour with no infection (Chimura *et al* 1993).

The cervical mucus also contains immunoglobulins. Although the mucus may act as a barrier to diffusion of large molecules, studies using fluorescence techniques to determine diffusion coefficients have demonstrated that immunoglobulins such as IgG, IgM and IgA diffuse almost as rapidly in cervical mucus as they do in water (Saltzman *et al* 1994). Plasma cells which secrete IgA have been demonstrated in the subepithelial layer of both the endocervix and ectocervix (Kutteh & Mestecky 1994). Secretory IgA can be detected in cervical mucus and a local specific immune response of this type can be demonstrated in some women where no evidence of any systemic immune response is present (Persson *et al* 1988).

Amniotic fluid

The amniotic fluid has antibacterial activity, which increases with gestation, particularly after 28 weeks (Bergman *et al* 1972, Jankowski *et al* 1977, Kalamaras *et al* 1980, Honkonen & Erikkola 1987).

The first bacterial growth inhibiting factor that was described was a low molecular weight peptide, which acts with zinc to form a zinc-peptide antibacterial system (Schleivert *et al* 1975, 1976). Synthesis of the peptide component seems to occur at around 20 weeks gestation but true antibacterial activity is obtained after this time, when the phosphate to zinc ratio of the fluid is low, because phosphate is inhibitory to the system (Schlievert *et al* 1977, Sachs & Stern 1979).

A high molecular weight component, beta lysin, has also been described, and both systems are dependent on divalent cations for their effective function (Ford *et al* 1981, Scane & Hawkins 1986). Other effectors of the antimicrobial activity of amniotic fluid include transferrin and lysozyme (Oka 1986, Oka 1987). Non-peptide antibacterial systems are also present; amniotic fluids with good in-vitro antibacterial activity have lower concentrations of bromide and potassium compared to those with poor activity (Honkonen *et al* 1986). Amniotic fluid also possesses immuno-modulatory activity. It can inhibit chlamydial inclusion body formation in McCoy cell cultures (Ismail *et al* 1991) and strongly inhibits the in-vitro generation of cell-mediated cytolytic responses to allogenic tumour cells in mice (Gambel *et al* 1982). Preincubation of polymorphonuclear leukocytes in amniotic fluid leads to decreased phagocytic activity and phagocytic index (Stefanovic *et al* 1993).

Several studies have shown that amniotic fluid has broad spectrum antibacterial activity (Sachs & Stern 1979, Scane & Hawkins 1984, Larsen *et al* 1984, Scane & Hawkins 1986, Nazir *et al* 1987). However, there are large variations in activity between population groups (Appelbaum *et al* 1977) and individuals (Roquet *et al* 1981), such that amniotic fluid from different women may be active against different organisms, or different strains of the same organism (Larsen *et al* 1983). It is therefore possible that women with low amniotic fluid antibacterial activity to the organisms to which they are exposed are more prone to intrauterine infection and preterm labour or preterm prelabour amniorrhexis. A study of 39 pregnancies at 27-35 weeks of gestation reported that the antibacterial activity of amniotic fluid from women in preterm labour who failed to respond to tocolysis and delivered preterm was significantly lower than in women who responded to tocolysis or pregnancies that were not complicated by preterm labour (Nazir *et al* 1987).

The amniotic fluid contains immunoglobulins, in particular IgA produced by the fetal urogenital system and amniotic membranes, and their concentration increases with gestational age (Cleveland *et al* 1991). Deficiencies of trace elements or nutrients may impair immune function (Chandra 1985, Chandra 1992). For example, prolonged deficiency of zinc, which acts on metalloenzyme systems and has membrane stabilising functions, may lead to reduced cell-mediated immunity (Sugarman 1983).

INFECTION AS A CAUSE OF PRETERM DELIVERY

There are essentially three causes of preterm delivery:

(i) Iatrogenic for maternal or fetal indications, such as pre-eclampsia, antepartum haemorrhage, or intrauterine growth retardation; in a small number of cases of intrauterine growth retardation the underlying cause is maternal-fetal infection with such organisms as toxoplasma, rubella virus, or cytomegalovirus,

(ii) Preterm prelabour amniorrhexis, where approximately 40% of the cases have evidence of intrauterine infection with organisms found in the lower genital tract, and

(iii) Preterm labour with intact membranes, where about one tenth of the cases have evidence of intrauterine infection with organisms found in the lower genital tract.

In preterm prelabour amniorrhexis, the evidence that infection may be the cause of subsequent preterm labour and delivery is based on the demonstration that in the group with intrauterine infection (i) spontaneous delivery occurs earlier than in those without infection, and (ii) there is increased amniotic fluid concentration of prostaglandins, leukotrienes and a variety of inflammatory mediators, that can induce uterine contractions.

Similarly, in patients with preterm labour and intact membranes, the amniotic fluid concentration of prostaglandins, leukotrienes and cytokines is higher in those with positive amniotic fluid cultures; in this group tocolytics are less successful in arresting labour than in those with no infection.

Interval from amniorrhexis to delivery

A study involving culture of amniotic fluid, obtained by amniocentesis from 110 patients with preterm prelabour amniorrhexis, reported that the median admission-to-delivery interval was significantly shorter in those cases with positive cultures (20 hours) compared to those with negative cultures (59 hours; Romero *et al* 1993). In another study, involving 221 patients with amniorrhexis that had amniocentesis, the incidence of positive amniotic fluid cultures was significantly higher in those presenting in labour (39%), compared to those that were not in labour (25%; Romero *et al* 1988a).

Carroll *et al* (1995b) reported a study of 69 pregnancies with preterm prelabour amniorrhexis at 12-36 weeks of gestation that were managed expectantly and had spontaneous onset of labour. In all cases cordocentesis and amniocentesis were performed and fetal blood and amniotic fluid were cultured for aerobic and anaerobic bacteria; the amniotic fluid was also cultured for *Mycoplasma* species. In the group with negative fetal blood and amniotic fluid cultures, the median interval from amniorrhexis to delivery was 41 days (range 1-161) and there was an inverse correlation between gestational age at amniorrhexis and the interval between amniorrhexis and delivery (Figure 2.1). In the group with negative fetal blood but positive amniotic fluid cultures (usually *Mycoplasma* species), the median amniorrhexis to delivery interval was nine days (range 1-37), and in the group with positive fetal blood cultures the interval was two days (range 1-5) (Figure 2.2).

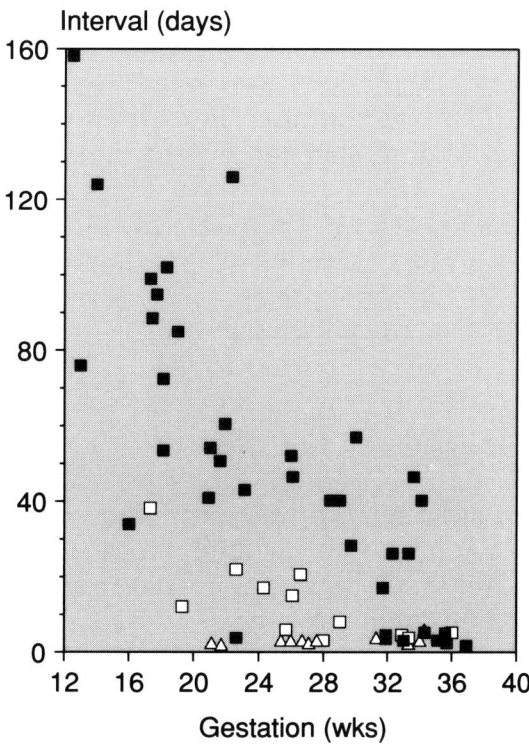

Figure 2.1. Time interval (days) between preterm prelabour amniorrhexis and spontaneous onset of labour in relation to gestation (weeks) at amniorrhexis in patients with negative fetal blood and amniotic fluid cultures (■), negative fetal blood but positive amniotic fluid cultures (□), and those with positive fetal blood cultures (△).

In patients with positive fetal blood and amniotic fluid cultures, the suggested mechanism for the association between infection and labour is release of cytokines which stimulate production of prostaglandins that induce uterine contractions. In the non-infected group, the finding of an inverse correlation between gestation at amniorrhexis and the latent period suggests that, with advancing gestation, there is an increase in uterine sensitivity to the trigger of labour which is not mediated by infection.

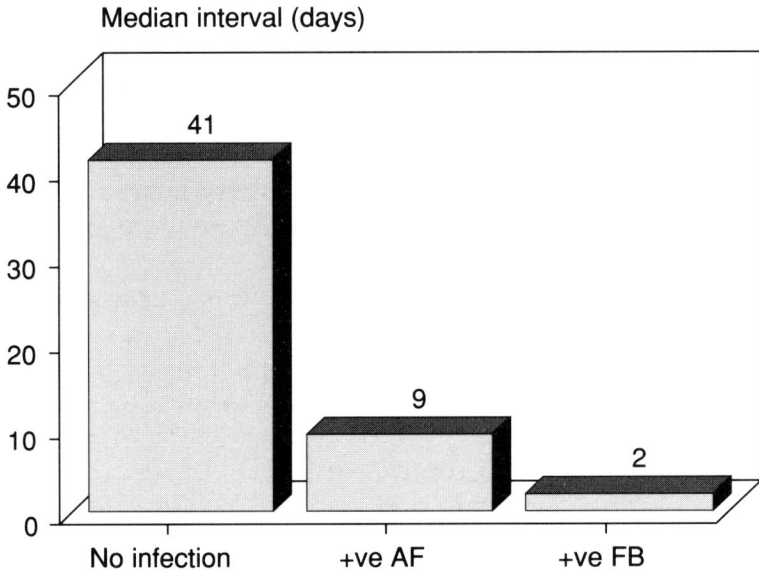

Median interval (days)

Figure 2.2. Median interval from amniorrhexis to delivery in patients with no intrauterine infection and those with positive amniotic fluid (AF) or positive fetal blood (FB) cultures. Adapted from Carroll *et al* (1995b).

Further support for infection as a mediator of preterm delivery is the finding that antibiotic therapy is associated with prolongation of the interval between amniorrhexis and delivery (see Chapter 4). However, this prolongation is only for a few days, suggesting that administration of antibiotics to the mother may not eradicate intrauterine infection but may merely achieve temporary reduction in the organism load. Alternatively, even if antibiotics do eradicate infection, they may not be able to interrupt the cascade of cytokine activation leading to labour and delivery.

Intrauterine infection, cytokines and prostaglandins

The suggested mechanism for the association between intra-uterine infection and labour is infection-mediated release of cytokines which stimulate production of prostaglandins that induce uterine contractions.

Prostaglandins and leukotrienes in normal labour

The chorioamniotic membranes contain the substrates and necessary enzymes for synthesis and degradation of prostaglandins and leukotrienes, which probably constitute the final mediator for the onset and maintenance of labour (Keirse & Turnbull 1975, 1976). Phospholipase enzymes act on membrane phospholipids to produce arachidonic acid, which can either be converted to prostaglandins, by the cyclo-oxygenase pathway, or into leukotrienes, by the lipoxygenase pathway (Figure 2.3).

With the onset and progress of labour, there is a dramatic increase in the expression of cyclo-oxygenase gene in amnion and chorion (Bennett *et al* 1992), increase in prostaglandin synthesis by the membranes (Lopez-Bernal *et al* 1987) and increase in the levels of prostaglandins in amniotic fluid (Keirse and Turnbull 1975). Furthermore, the administration of exogenous prostaglandins increases uterine activity, whereas prostaglandin synthase inhibitors can suppress labour (Zuckerman *et al* 1974, Novy & Liggins 1980, Okazaki *et al* 1981).

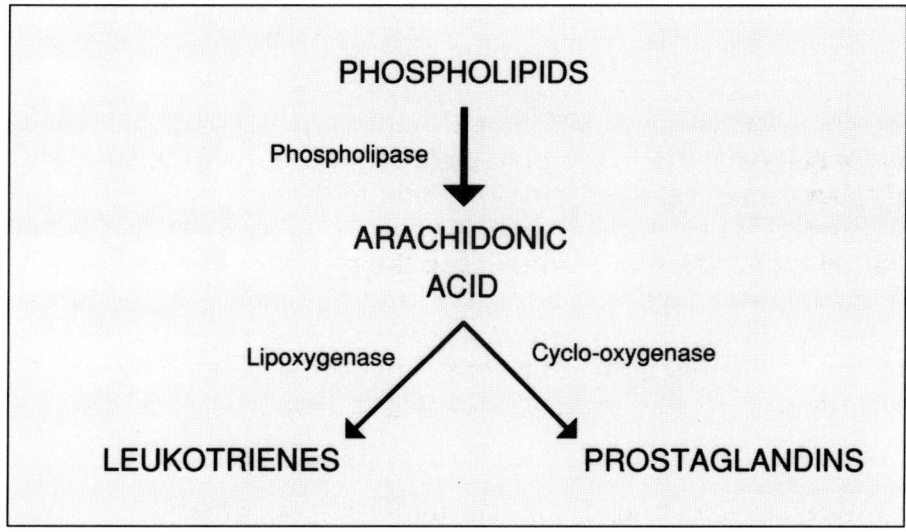

Figure 2.3. Arachidonic acid metabolism.

In addition to prostaglandins, labour at term is associated with increased membrane production and amniotic fluid concentration of leukotrienes (Bernal *et al* 1990, Romero *et al* 1988c, Walsh 1989). However, this increase is not observed after preterm labour, unless there is associated chorioamnionitis. These findings suggest that maturation of the lipoxygenase pathway occurs towards term and the maturational process is altered by inflammation.

The membranes also produce cytokines, but the physiological significance of these substances in normal labour remains unclear. It may be that some of the mediators which are classically associated with inflammation or infection play key roles in the initiation of normal human parturition (Pasetto *et al* 1993).

Bacteria-induced preterm delivery

Intrauterine infection, either directly or through the host response (cytokines), may stimulate amniotic membranes to synthesise prostaglandins that induce uterine contractions.

In vitro studies have demonstrated that the various organisms involved in intrauterine infection produce phospholipases which are able to stimulate prostaglandin release from cultured amnion cells; prostaglandin production is also stimulated by various endotoxins (Bejar *et al* 1981, Bennett *et al* 1987, Romero *et al* 1988d, Lamont *et al* 1990). Furthermore, in-vitro studies have demonstrated that, although production of prostaglandins by membranes is higher after term than preterm delivery, the highest production is observed in the presence of chorioamnionitis (Table 2.6; Lopez-Bernal *et al* 1987, 1989).

Table 2.6. Prostaglandin E (PGE) production by amnion (fmol/mg dry weight per two hours) after term and preterm delivery with and without histological evidence of chorioamnionitis (Lopez-Bernal *et al* 1989).

Metabolite	PGE
Preterm delivery with no chorioamnionitis	1,414
Preterm delivery with chorioamnionitis	12,278
Term delivery with no chorioamnionitis	2,640

Cytokines, such as interleukins 1, 6 and 8, produced in response to inflammation, can stimulate activation of the lipoxygenase and cyclo-oxygenase pathways, leading to production of many arachidonic acid metabolites that induce labour. For example, recent molecular biology studies have demonstrated that interleukin-1 (IL-1) stimulates specific receptors on amnion to induce production of cyclo-oxygenase II; specific mRNA for the enzyme was demonstrated within 30 minutes of stimulation (Mitchell *et al* 1993). Amnion cells, like other epithelial cells, respond to stimulation by one cytokine to produce other cytokines. For example, IL-1β stimulates cultured amnion cells to produce IL-8 mRNA (Trautman *et al* 1992).

Microbial invasion of the amniotic fluid and/or preterm labour are associated with increased concentrations of prostaglandins, leukotrienes and a variety of inflammatory mediators (Table 2.7).

Table 2.7. Median amniotic fluid concentration of arachidonic acid metabolites and cytokines in preterm prelabour amniorrhexis or in preterm labour with intact membranes in the presence of positive or negative amniotic fluid cultures (AF).

Metabolite	Author	Labour		No labour	
		AF+ve	AF -ve	AF+ve	AF -ve
PGE2 (pg/mL)	Romero *et al* 1987a	3,143	290	502	278
PGF2 (pg/mL)	Romero *et al* 1987a	2,649	183	340	187
PGF2 (pg/mL)	Romero *et al* 1989a	720	87	-	-
PGFM (pg/mL)	Romero *et al* 1989a	1,390	510	-	-
PGEM II (pg/mL)	Romero *et al* 1989a	4,143	1,485	-	-
12 HETE (μg/mL)	Romero *et al* 1987b	15	10	10	6
15 HETE (ng/mL)	Romero *et al* 1987b	1,817	386	677	200
5 HETE (ng/mL)	Romero *et al* 1988b	1,876	2,052	-	-
LTB4 (pg/mL)	Romero *et al* 1987b	98	10	16	0
TNF (pg/mL)	Romero *et al* 1992a	249	<60	<60	<60
TNF (pg/mL)	Hillier *et al* 1993	400	0	-	-
TNF (pg/mL)	Romero *et al* 1989b	750	<200	-	-
IL-1 (iu/mL)	Romero *et al* 1989c	100	<1	<1	<1
IL-1α (pg/mL)	Hillier *et al* 1993	175	0	-	-
IL-1β (pg/mL)	Hillier *et al* 1993	250	0	-	-
IL-1β (iu/mL)	Carroll *et al* 1995c	-	-	33	19
IL-6 (pg/mL)	Hillier *et al* 1993	9,500	2,000	-	-
IL-6 (pg/mL)	Greig *et al* 1993	2,592	153		
IL-8 (ng/mL)	Romero *et al* 1991b	80	<0.3	-	-
IL-8 (ng/mL)	Cherouny *et al* 1993	64	<1	-	-
Endothelin (fmol/mL)	Romero *et al* 1992	150	62	-	-

PG = Prostaglandin, HETE = Hydroxyeicosatetraenoic acid, LT = Leukotriene,
TNF=Tumour necrosis factor, IL = Interleukin

The highest concentrations are observed in cases with both infection and labour.

Carroll *et al* (1995c) measured IL-1β concentration in fetal and maternal plasma and amniotic fluid from pregnancies complicated by preterm prelabour amniorrhexis. In patients with positive fetal blood and/or amniotic fluid cultures, plasma and amniotic fluid levels of IL-1β were higher (Figure 2.4) and the interval between amniorrhexis and onset of labour was shorter than in the non-infected group. However, there were no significant associations between fetal plasma IL-1β and maternal plasma or amniotic fluid IL-1β, fetal leukocyte count or the interval between amniorrhexis and the onset of labour.

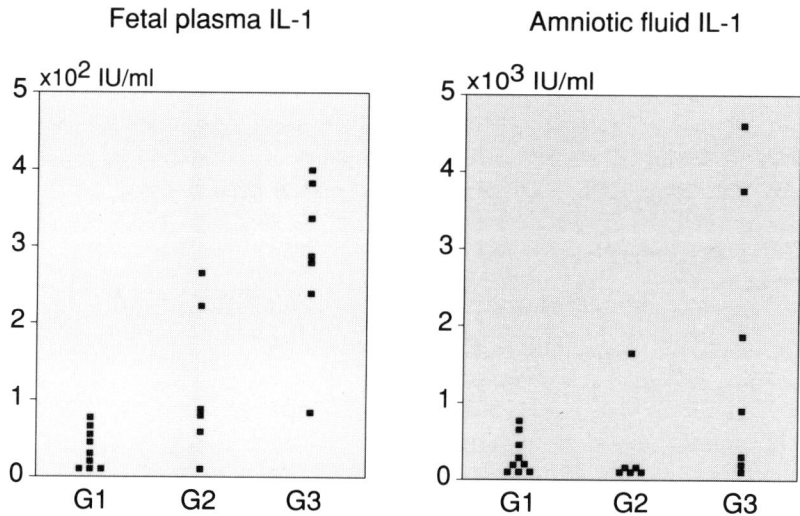

Figure 2.4. Fetal plasma and amniotic fluid interleukin-1β concentration (IL-1) in pregnancies complicated by preterm prelabour amniorrhexis (group 1 = no infection, group 2 = microbial invasion of the amniotic cavity, group 3 = fetal bacteraemia). Adapted from Carroll et al (1995c).

The lack of significant association between fetal plasma and amniotic fluid IL-1β concentrations does not preclude a common source of IL-1β; findings in a cross-sectional study do not allow conclusions to be drawn on the dynamic interrelation between two biological compartments. Since in the infected group the maternal plasma IL-1β concentration was not increased, it is unlikely that transplacental transfer from the mother can explain the findings in fetal plasma and amniotic fluid. Similarly, the lack of significant association between fetal leukocyte count and fetal plasma IL-1β does not exclude fetal leukocytes as the source of IL-1β; fetal infection is associated with changes in lymphocyte subpopulations in the presence of normal leukocyte counts (Thilaganathan *et al* 1994).

The lack of a significant association between fetal plasma or amniotic fluid IL-1β concentrations and the interval between amniorrhexis and onset of labour is in apparent contradiction with the hypothesis that there is a direct causal association between infection, cytokines, prostaglandins and labour. However, the lack of a statistical association between cytokine concentration and delivery interval in a cross-sectional study does not rule out a role for cytokines in the initiation of labour. The temporal relationship between infection, cytokines and prostaglandins can only be explored by serial sampling of amniotic fluid.

In a study on chronically instrumented pregnant rhesus monkeys, intra-amniotic inoculation of group B streptococcus was performed on day 130 of gestation (Figure 2.5; Gravett *et al* 1994).

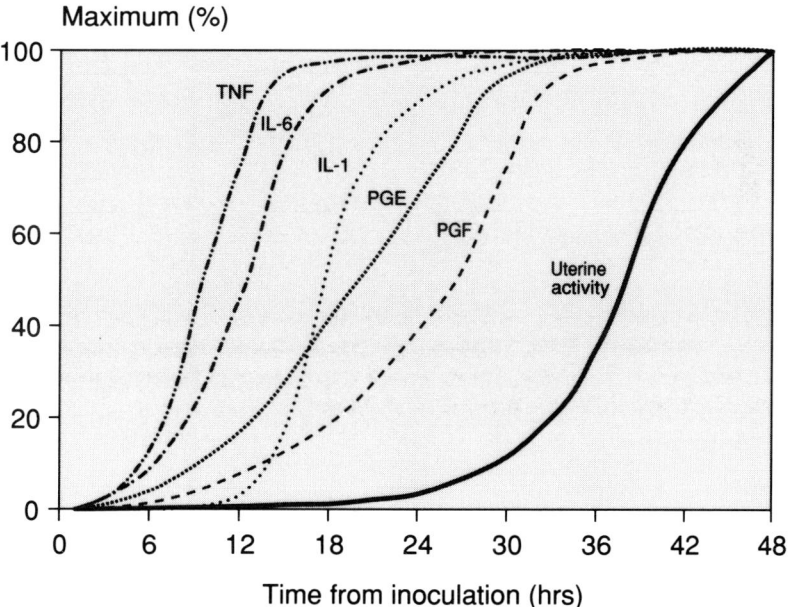

Figure 2.5. Temporal relationship between increase in amniotic fluid concentration of cytokines and prostaglandins and onset of labour following intra-amniotic inoculation of bacteria. Adapted from Gravett *et al* (1994).

About 10-20 hours after inoculation, there was an increase in amniotic fluid concentration of tumour necrosis factor and then interleukins 6 and 1. About six hours after the initial increase in cytokines, there was a rise in the concentration of prostaglandins E and F. Finally, there was an increase in uterine activity about 30 hours after the inoculation. This study also demonstrated that the peak amniotic fluid concentration of prostaglandins in the monkeys with iatrogenic intra-amniotic infection was seven times higher than in those undergoing spontaneous labour at term without infection.

INTRAUTERINE INFECTION AND RISK OF NEONATAL SEPSIS

Diagnosis of neonatal sepsis

The diagnosis of neonatal sepsis is based on the demonstration of a positive blood or cerebrospinal fluid culture. The latter is necessary in all neonates with suspected sepsis because cerebrospinal fluid cultures may be positive in up to 15% of cases with negative blood cultures (Visser & Hall 1980). Urine cultures may also be performed but these are more useful in the detection of acquired, rather than congenital sepsis and have a low yield if performed within the first 72 hours after birth (Visser & Hall 1979).

Possible neonatal sepsis

Mortality from neonatal sepsis is very high and therefore antibiotic therapy is often necessary before the results of cultures are available. Consequently, therapy is instituted on the basis of the clinical condition of the neonate and the results of a series of rapid tests (Table 2.8).

Neonatal sepsis is associated with neutropenia, leukopenia and thrombocytopenia, but the number of immature leukocytes is increased. Infection is also associated with increased erythrocyte sedimentation rate and increased concentrations of C-reactive protein and products of complement, such as C3d.

Table 2.8. True positive rate (TP) and false positive rate (FP) of various haematological indices in the prediction of neonatal sepsis. Adapted from Gerdes (1991).

Test	TP	FP
Leukocyte count (<5,000/mm³)	29%	9%
Neutrophil count (<1,750/mm³)	38-96%	8-39%
Platelet count (<150,000/ mm³)	22-38%	1-18%
Toxic granulation of leukocytes	67-81%	7-10%
Immature to total neutrophil ratio (>0.2)	90-100%	22-50%
Erythrocyte sedimentation rate raised	27-50%	3-17%
C-reactive protein (>1mg/dl)	47-100%	6-17%
Complement products present (C3d)	74%	16%

Incidence of neonatal sepsis

The incidence of neonatal sepsis in the general population is about 0.1-0.8% (Gerdes 1991). In patients with preterm prelabour amniorrhexis, the risk of neonatal sepsis is about 10 times higher than in the general population and the risk is increased four-fold in those with positive amniotic fluid cultures compared to those with negative cultures (Table 2.9, Figure 2.6).

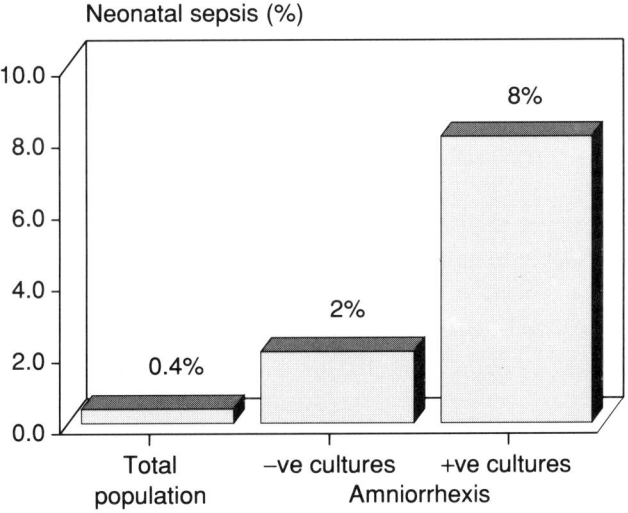

Figure 2.6. Incidence of neonatal sepsis in the total population and in pregnancies with preterm prelabour amniorrhexis and positive or negative amniotic fluid cultures.

Table 2.9. Incidence of neonatal sepsis (positive blood and / or cerebrospinal fluid cultures) in patients with preterm prelabour amniorrhexis. Some of the studies also give the incidence of neonatal sepsis in relation to the results of amniotic fluid culture.

Author	N	Incidence of neonatal sepsis		
		Total	Amniotic fluid culture	
			Positive	Negative
Seo *et al* 1992	306	8%	-	-
Miller *et al* 1978	151	7%	-	-
Thibeault & Emmanouilides 1977	153	3%	-	-
Daikoku *et al* 1981	203	1%	-	-
Roussis *et al* 1991	99	4%	-	-
Wilson *et al* 1982	145	7%	-	-
Kappy *et al* 1979	188	1%	-	-
Alger *et al* 1988	52	0%	-	-
Broekhuizen *et al* 1985	88	4%	6%	3%
Cotton *et al* 1984	61	5%	16%	3%
Bengston *et al* 1989	61	2%	-	-
Blott & Greenough 1988	30	6%	-	-
Romero *et al* 1993	110	4%	5%	3%
Gauthier *et al* 1992	111	1%	0%	2%
Garite & Freeman 1982	86	8%	15%	3%
Coultrip & Grossman 1992	29	7%	17%	0%
Vintzileos *et al* 1986	54	7%	33%	0%
Fayez *et al* 1978	53	4%	-	-
Total	**1,980**	**5%**	**8%**	**2 %**

The incidence of neonatal sepsis in pregnancies with preterm prelabour amniorrhexis and in those with preterm labour and intact membranes is inversely related to gestational age (Figure 2.7).

The most common organisms implicated in neonatal sepsis are *Escherichia coli, Klebsiella, Enterobacter, Pseudomonas, Serratia marcescans, Streptococcus agalactiae, Streptococcus pneumoniae, Staphylococcus aureus, Staphylococcus epidermidis, Haemophilus influenzae, Bacteroides, Gardnerella vaginalis* and *Candida albicans* (Siegel & McCracken 1981, Ohlsson & Vearncombe 1987, Day *et al* 1992, Thompson *et al* 1992).

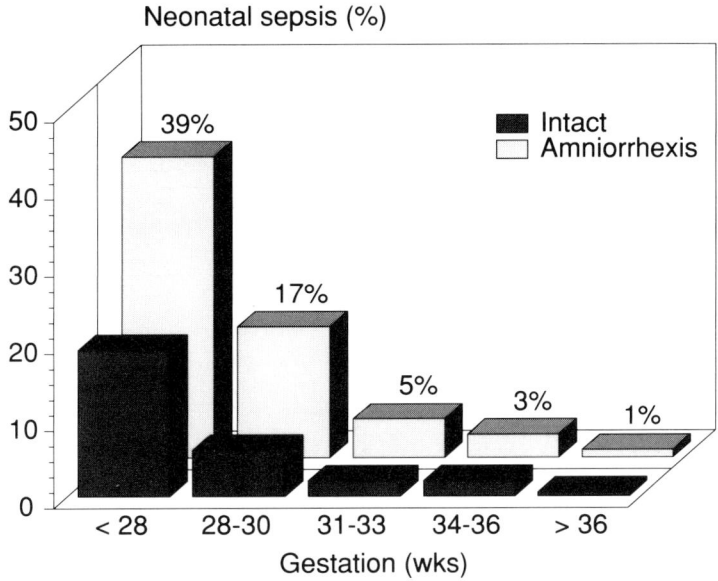

Figure 2.7. Incidence of neonatal sepsis in pregnancies with preterm prelabour amniorrhexis and in those with preterm labour and intact membranes in relation to gestational age. Adapted from Seo *et al* (1992).

Neonatal sepsis in patients with preterm prelabour amniorrhexis is most probably acquired in utero rather than during delivery. Supporting evidence is provided by the finding that the incidence of neonatal sepsis in pregnancies with positive amniotic fluid cultures is much higher than in the general population, despite the fact that the incidence of colonisation of the lower genital tract with pathogens is similar in patients with preterm prelabour amniorrhexis and in those with no pregnancy complications (see Chapter 3). Nevertheless, it is possible that in patients with amniorrhexis the virulence of organisms in the lower genital tract is greater, and in this respect it is possible that, at least in some cases of neonatal sepsis, the infection is acquired during delivery. Ultimately, this issue can only be resolved by randomised trials examining the incidence of neonatal sepsis in relation to mode of delivery. In the meantime, there is some evidence that, in patients with positive lower genital tract cultures for *Streptococcus agalactiae*, intrapartum treatment with antibiotics reduces the incidence of neonatal sepsis; in a randomised study the incidence of sepsis in the treated group was 0%, compared to 6% for the controls (Boyer *et al* 1986).

Mortality from neonatal sepsis

The reported mortality rate in neonates with congenital systemic bacterial infection varies from 25% to 90% (Placzek & Whitelaw 1983, Boyer *et al* 1983, Ohlsson & Vearncombe 1987, Gerdes 1991, Thompson *et al* 1992). However, there is a sparsity of studies comparing mortality in infected neonates to controls matched for gestation at delivery and birth weight. One such study that examined 168 infants born at less than 33 weeks of gestation reported that the mortality in the infected group was 33% compared to 17% for those that were not infected (Thompson *et al* 1992). Furthermore, neonatal mortality is higher in those with congenital rather than postnatally acquired sepsis (Ohlsson & Vearncombe 1987).

CONCLUSION

Current evidence suggests that intrauterine infection is the cause rather than the consequence of amniorrhexis. In about 10% of pregnancies with preterm labour and intact membranes and in 40% of those with preterm prelabour amniorrhexis, the amniotic fluid cultures are positive with organisms commonly found in the lower genital tract. The main adverse sequelae of intrauterine infection are preterm delivery and neonatal sepsis.

REFERENCES

Alger LS, Lovchik JC, Hebel JR, Blackmon LR, Crenshaw MC. The association of chlamydia trachomatis, neisseria gonorrhoeae and group B streptococci with preterm PROM and pregnancy outcome. Am J Obstet Gynecol 1988;159:397-404.

Appelbaum PC, Holloway Y, Ross SM, Dhupelia I. The effect of amniotic fluid on bacterial growth in three population groups. Am J Obstet Gynecol 1977;128:868-71.

Bakowski B, Tschesche H. Migration of polymorphonuclear leukocytes through human amnion membranes-a scanning electron microscopic study. Biol Chem Hoppe Seyler 1992 Jun;373;7:529-46.

Bejar R, Curbelo V, Davis C, Gluck L. Premature labour.II. Bacterial sources of phospholipase. Obstet Gynecol 1981;57:479-82.

Bengston JM, Van Marter LJ, Barss VA, Greene MF, Tuomala RE, Epstein MF. Pregnancy outcome after premature rupture of the membranes at or before 26 weeks gestation. Obstet Gynecol 1989;73:921-6.

Bennett PR, Henderson DJ, Moore GE. Changes in the expression of the cyclooxygenase gene in human fetal membranes and placenta with labour. Am J Obstet Gynecol 1992;167:212-16.

Bennett PR, Rose MP, Myatt L, Elder MG. Preterm labour:stimulation of arachidonic acid metabolism in human amnion cells by bacterial products. Am J Obstet Gynecol1987;156:649-55.

Bergman N, Bercovici B, Sacks T. Antibacterial activity of human amniotic fluid. Am J Obstet Gynecol 1972;114;4:520-3.

Bernal AL, Hansell DJ, Khong TY, Keeling JW, Turnbull AC. Placental leukotriene B4 release in early pregnancy and in term and preterm labour. Early Hum Dev 1990;23:93-9.

Blott M, Greenough A. Neonatal outcome after prolonged rupture of the membranes starting in the second trimester. Arch Dis Child 1988;63:1146-50.

Boyer KM, Gadzala chorioamnionitis, Burd LI, Fisher DE, Paton JB, Gotoff SP. Selective intrapartum chemoprophylaxis of neonatal group B streptococcual early onset disease.I.Epidemiologic rationalle. J Inf Dis 1983;148:795-801.

Boyer KM, Gotoff SP. Prevention of early onset neonatal group B streptococcal disease with selective intrapartum chemoprophylaxis. NEJM 1986;314:1665-9.

Broekhuizen FF, Gilman M, Hamilton PR. Amniocentesis for Gram stain and culture in preterm premature rupture of the membranes. Obstet Gynecol 1985;66:316-21.

Carroll SG, Papaioannou S, Ntumazah IL, Philpott-Howard J, Nicolaides KH. Lower genital tract swabs in the prediction of intrauterine infection in preterm prelabour amniorrhexis. Br J Obstet Gynaecol 1995a (In press).

Carroll SG, Ville Y, Greenough A, Gamsu H, Patel B, Philpott-Howard J, Nicolaides KH. Preterm prelabour amniorrhexis: intrauterine infection and interval between membrane rupture and delivery. Arch Dis Child 1995b;72: F43-6.

Carroll SG, Abbas A, Ville Y, Meher-Homjii H, Nicolaides KH. Fetal plasma and amniotic fluid interleukin-1 concentration in pregnancies complicated by preterm prelabour amniorrhexis. J Clin Path 1995c (In press).

Chandra RK. Grace A goldsmith award lecture. trace element regulation of immunity and infection. J Am Coll Nutr 1985;4;1:5-16.

Chandra RK. Nutrition and immunoregulation. Significance for host resistance to tumours and infectious diseases in humans and rodents. J Nutr 1992 Mar;122;3:754-7.

Cherouny PH, Pankuch GA, Romero R, Botti JJ, Kuhn DC, Demers LM, Appelbaum PC. Neutrophil attractant/activating peptide-1/interleukin-8:Association with histologic chorioamnionitis, preterm delivery and bioactive fluid leukoattractants.Am J Obstet Gynecol 1993;169:1299-303.

Chimura T, Hirayama T, Takase M. Lysozyme in cervical mucus in patients with chorioamnionitis. Jpn J Antibiot 1993;46:726-9.

Cleveland MG, Bakos MA, Pyron DL, Rajaraman S, Goldblum RM. Characterisation of secretory component in amniotic fluid: identification of new forms of secretory IgA. J Immunol 1991;147;1:181-8.

Cotton DB, Hill LM, Strassner HT, Platt LD, Ledger WJ. Use of amniocentesis in preterm gestation with ruptured membranes. Obstet Gynecol 1984;63:38-48.

Coultrip LL, Grossman JH. Evaluation of rapid diagnostic tests in the detection of microbial invasion of the amniotic cavity. Am J Obstet Gynecol 1992;167:1231-42.

Daikoku NH, Kaltreider F, Johnson TRB, Johnson JWC, Simmons MA. Premature rupture of membranes and preterm labour: Neonatal infection and perinatal mortality risks. Obstet Gynecol 1981;58:417-25.

Day D, Ugol JH, French JI, Haverkamp A, Wall RE, McGregor JA. Fetal monitoring in perinatal sepsis. Am J Perinatol 1992;9:28-33.

Dillon HC, Khare S, Gray BM. Group B streptococcal carriage and disease: A 6 year prospective study. J Pediatr 1987;110:31-6.

Dudley J, Malcolm G, Ellwood D. Amniocentesis in the mamagement of preterm premature rupture of the membranes. Aust NZ J Obstet Gynaecol 1991;31:331-6.

Dunlow SG, Duff P. Microbiology of the lower genital tract and amniotic fluid in asymptomatic preterm patients with intact membranes and moderate to advanced degrees of cervical effacement and dilation. Am J Perinatol 1990;7:235-8.

Easterling A, Burton GJ, Skepper JN, Nasr-Esfahani MH. A scanning electron microscopic study of the chick chorioallantoic membrane: cell death and the involvement of oxygen free radicals. Scanning Microsc 1993;7:87-95.

Evaldson GR, Larsson B, Jiborn H. Is the collagen content reduced when the fetal membranes rupture? Gynecol Obstet Invest 1987;24:92-4.

Fayez JA, Hasan AA, Jona HS, Miller GL. Management of premature rupture of the membranes. Obstet Gynecol 1978;52:17-21.

Fisk NM, Fysh J, Child AG, Gatenby PA, Jeffery H, Bradfield AH. Is C-reactive protein really useful in preterm premature rupture of the membranes. Br J Obstet Gynaecol 1987;94:1159-64.

Ford LC, Lagasse LD, Kasha W, Heins Y, DeLange RJ, Wright JD, Alexander G, Lebhertz TB. Identification of beta lysin as a zinc dependent protein in amniotic fluid. J Obstet Gynaecol 1981;2:79-84.

Galask RP, Varner MW, Petzold R, Wilbur SL. Attachment to the chorioamniotic membranes. Am J Obstet Gynecol 1984;148:915-25.

Gambel PI, Ferguson FG. Suppression of cellular immune responses by mouse amniotic fluid. J Clin Lab Immunol 1982;8:203-5.

Garite TJ, Freeman RK. Chorioamnionitis in the preterm gestation. Obstet Gynecol 1982;59:539-45.

Gauthier DW, Meyer WJ, Bieniarz A. Biophysical profile as a predictor of amniotic fluid culture results. Obstet Gynecol 1992; 80:102-5.

Gauthier DW, Meyer WJ, Bieniarz A. Correlation of amniotic fluid glucose concentration and intraamniotic infection in patients with preterm labour or premature rupture of membranes. Am J Obstet Gynecol 1991;165:1105-61.

Gerdes JS. Clinicopathologic approach to the diagnosis of neonatal sepsis. Clin Perinat 1991;18:361-81.

Gravett MG, Hummel D, Eschenbach DA, Holmes KK. Preterm labour associated with subclinical amniotic fluid infection and with bacterial vaginosis. Obstet Gynecol 1986;67:229-36.

Gravett MG, Witkin SS, Haluska GJ, Edwards JL, Cook MJ, Novy MJ. An Experimental model for intraamniotic infection and preterm labour in rhesus monkeys. Am J Obstet Gynecol 1994;171:1660-7.

Greig PC, Ernest JM, Teot L, Erikson M, Talley R. Amniotic fluid interleukin-6 levels correlate with histological chorioamnionitis and amniotic fluid cultures in patients in premature labour with intact membranes. Am J Obstet Gynecol 1993;169:1035-44.

Guzick DS, Winn K. The association of chorioamnionitis with preterm delivery. Obstet Gynecol 1985;65:11-15.

Gyr TN, Malek A, Mathez-Loic F, Altermatt HJ, Bodmer T, Nicolaides K, Schneider H. Permeation of human chorioamniotic membranes by Escherichia coli in vitro. Am J Obstet Gynecol 1994;170:223-7.

Hay PE, Lamont RF, Taylor-Robinson D, Morgan DJ, Ison C, Pearson J. Abnormal bacterial colonisation of the genital tract and subsequent preterm delivery and late miscarriage. BMJ 1994;308:295-8.

Heddleston L, McDuffie RS, Gibbs RS. A rabbit model for ascending infection in preganncy: Intervention with indomethacin and delayed ampicillin-sulbactam therapy. Am J Obstet Gynecol 1993;169:708-12.

Hillier SL, Martius J, Krohn M, Kiviat N, Holmes KK, Eschenbach DA. A case control study of chorioamniotic infection and histologic chorioamnionitis in prematurity. NEJM 1988;972-7.

Hillier SL, Witkin SS, Krohn MA, Watts DH, Kiviat NB, Eschenbach DA. The relationship of amniotic fluid cytokines and preterm delivery, amniotic fluid infection, histologic chorioamnionitis and chorioamnion infection. Obstet Gynecol 1993;81:941-8.

Honkonen E, Erikkola R. Antibacterialcapacity in amniotic fluid in normal and complicated pregnancies. Ann Chir Gynaecol Suppl 1987;202:14-16.

Honkonen E, Nanto V, Hyora H, Vuorinen K, Erkkola R. Trace elements and antibacterial activity in amniotic fluid. Biol Neonate1986;50;1:21-6.

Ismail MA, Salti GI, Block BS, Moawad AH. The effect of filtration of amniotic fluid on the growth of Chlamydia trachomatis and Escherichia coli. Am J Perinatol 1991;8;1:50-2.

Ismail MA, Zinaman MJ, Lowensohn RI, Moawad AH. The significance of C-reactive protein levels in women with premature rupture of the membranes . Am J Obstet Gynecol 1985;151:541-4.

Jankowski RP, Aikins HE, Vahrson H, Gupta KG. Antibacterial activity of amniotic fluid against staphylococcus aureus, candida albicans and brucella abortus. Arch Gynakol 1977;222:275-8.

Kalamaras E, Karanfislka N, Dzikov Z, Kalamaras A. The effect of amniotic fluid on bacteria. Jugosl Ginekol Obstet. 1980;19:139-44.

Kanayama N, Terao T, Kawashima Y, Horiuchi K, Fujimoto D. Collagen types in normal and prematurely ruptured amniotic membranes. Am J Obstet Gynecol1985;153:899-903.

Kappy KA, Cetrulo CL, Knuppel RA, Ingardia CJ, Sbarra AJ, Scerbo JC, Mitchell GW. Premature rupture of the membranes: A conservative approach. Am J Obstet Gynecol 1979;134:655-61.

Keirse MJNC, Turnbull AC. Metabolism of prostaglandins within the pregnant uterus. Br J Obstet Gynaecol 1975;82:887-93.

Keirse MJNC, Turnbull AC. The fetal membranes as a possible source of amniotic fluid prostaglandins. Br J Obstet Gynaecol 1976;83:146-51.

Kitajima H, Nakayama M, Miyano A, Shimizu, Taniguchi T, Shimoya K, Matsuzaki N, Fujimura. Significance of chorioamnionitis. Early Hum Dev 1992;29:125-30.

Klima G, Schmidt W. Immunohistochemical studies of the nature of connective tissue in fetal membranes. Acta Histochem 1988;84:195-203.

Klima G, Zerlauth B, Richter J, Schmidt W. The microtexture of amnion and chorion connective tissue. Anat Anz 1989;168:395-400.

Kurki T, Sivonen A, Renkonen O, Savia E, Ylikorkala O. Bacterial vaginosis in early pregnancy and pregnancy outcome. Obstet Gynecol 1992;80:173-7.

Kutteh WH, Mestecky J. Secretory immunity in the female reproductive tract. Am J Reprod Immunol 1994;31:40-6.

Lamont RF, Anthony F, Myatt L, Booth L, Furr PM, Taylor-Robinson D. Production of prostaglandin E2 by human amnion in vitro in response to addition of media conditioned by micoorganisms associated with chorioamnionitis and preterm labour. Am J Obstet Gynecol 1990;162:819-25.

Lamont RF, Rose MP, Elder MG. Effect of bacterial products on prostaglandin E production by amnion cells. Lancet 1985;2:331-3.

Larsen B, Davis B, Charles D. Critical assessment of antibacterial properties of human amniotic fluid. Gynecol Obstet Invest. 1984;18:100-4.

Larsen B, Hurrey DJ, Miro RE, Charles D. Antibacterial activity in amniotic fluid from west virginia women. Gynecol Obstet Invest 1983;15:26-32.

Lavery JP, Miller CE. Deformation and creep in the human chorioamniotic sac. Am J Obstet Gynecol 1979;134:366-75.

Leigh J, Garite TJ. Amniocentesis in the management of premature labour. Obstet Gynecol 1986;67:500-6.

Lopez-Bernal A, Hansell DJ, Khong TY, Keeling JW, Turnbull AC. Prostaglandin E production by the fetal membranes in unexplained preterm labour associated with chorioamnionitis. Br J Obstet Gynaecol 1989;96:1133-9.

Lopez-Bernal A, Hansell DJ, Soler RC, Keling JW, Turnbull AC. Prostaglandins, chorioamnionitis and preterm labour. Br J Obstet Gynaecol 1987;94:1156-8.

Major CA, Kitzmiller JL. Perinatal survival with expectant management of midtrimester rupture of membranes. Am J Obstet Gynecol 1990;163:838-44.

Malak TM, Bell SC. Structural characteristics of term human fetal membranes: a novel zone of extreme morphological alteration within the rupture site. Br J Obstet Gynaecol 1994;101:375-86.

Maxwell GL, Watson WJ. Preterm premature rupture of membranes: results of expectant management in patients with cervical cultures positive for group B streptococcus or Neisseria gonorrhoeae. Am J Obstet Gynecol1992;166:945-9.

McDonald HM, O'Loughlin JA, Jolley P, Vigneswaran R, McDonald PJ. Vaginal infection and preterm labour. Br J Obstet Gynecol 1991;98:427-35.

McGregor JA, French JI, Lawellin D, Franco-Buff A, Smith C, Todd JK. Bacterial protease induced reduction of chorioamniotic membrane strength and elasticity. Obstet Gynecol 1987;69:167-72.

McGregor JA, French JI, Seo K. Premature rupture of membranes and bacterial vaginosis. Am J Obstet Gynecol 1993;169:463-6.

McGregor JA, Lawellin D, Franco-Buff A, Todd JA, Makowski EL. Protease production by microorganisms associated with reproductive tract infection. Am J Obstet Gynecol 1986;154:109-14.

Meyer BA, Dickinson JE, Chambers C, Parisi VM. The effect of fetal sepsis on umbilical cord blood gases. Am J Obstet Gynecol 1992;166:612-17.

Miller JM, Pupkin MJ, Crenshaw C. Premature labour and preterm rupture of the membranes. Am J Obstet Gynecol 1978;132:1-6.

Mitchell MD, Edwin SS, Lundin-Schiller S, Silver RM, Smotkin D, Trautman MS. Mechanism of interleukin-1 beta stimulation of human amnion prostaglandin biosynthesis:mediation via a novel inducible cyclooxygenase. Placenta 1993;14:615-25.

Moretti M, Sibai BM. Maternal and perinatal outcome of expectant management of premature rupture of membranes in the midtrimester. Am J Obstet Gynecol 1988;159:390-6.

Mueller-Heubach E, Rubinstein DN, Schwarz SS. Histologic chorioamnionitis and preterm delivery in different patient populations. Obstet Gynecol 1990;75:622-5.

Nazir MA, Pankuch GA, Botti JJ, Appelbaum PC. Antibacterial activity of amniotic fluid in the early third trimester. Its association with preterm labour and delivery. Am J Perinatol 1987;4:59-62.

Newton ER, Clark M. Group B streptococcus and preterm rupture of membranes. Obstet Gynecol 1988;71:198-202.

Novy JM Liggins GC. Role of prostaglandins, prostacyclin and thromboxanes in the physiologic control of the uterus and in parturition. Sem Perin 1980;4:45-66.

O'Brien WF, Knuppel RA, Morales WJ, Angel JL, Torres CT. Amniotic fluid alpha 1-antitrypsin concentration in premature rupture of the membranes. Am J Obstet Gynecol 1990;162:756-9.

Ohlsson A, Vearncombe M. Congenital and nosocomial sepsis in infants born in a regional perinatal unit: Cause, outcome, and white blood cell response. Am J Obstet Gynecol 1987;156:407-13.

Oka K, Hagio Y, Tetsuoh M, Kawano K, Hamada T, Kato T. The effect of transferrin and lysozyme on antibacterial activity of amniotic fluid. Biol Res Pregnancy Perinatol 1987;8;1:1-6.

Oka K. A study on the antibacterial activity of amniotic fluid.The significance og intraamniotic transferrin. Nippon Sanka Fujinka Gakkai Zasshi 1986;38:461-9.

Okazaki T, Casey ML, Okita JR, MacDonald PC, Johnston JM. Initiation of human parturition.XII. Biosythesis and metabolism of prostaglandins in human fetal membranes and uterine decidua. Am J Obstet Gynecol 1981;139:373-81.

Pankuch GA, Appelbaum PC, Lorenz RP, Botti JJ, Schachter J, Naeye RL. Placental microbiology and histology and the pathogenesis of chorioamnionitis. Obstet Gynecol 1984;64:802-6.

Parmley TH. Spontaneous cell death in the chorion laeve. Am J Obstet Gynecol 1990;162:1576-83.

Pasetto N, Piccione E, Zicari A, Fontana L, DeCarolis C, Perricone R, Pontieri G, Ticconi C. Short report: cytokine production by human fetal membranes and uterine decidua at term gestation in relation to labour. Placenta 1993;14:361-4.

Persson E, Eneroth P, Jeansson S. Secretory IgA against herpes simplex virus in cervical secretions. Genitourin Med. 1988;64:373-7.

Pierce JR, Merenstein GB, Stocker JT. Immediate postmortem cultures in an intensive care nursery. Pediatr Inf Dis 1984;3:510-12

Placzek MM, Whitelaw A. Early and late neonatal septicemia. Arch Dis Child 1983;58:728-31.

Quinn PA, Butany J, Taylor J, Hannah W. Chrioamnionitis: Its association with pregnancy outcome and microbial infection. Am J Obstet Gynecol 1987;156:379-87.

Romero R, Emamian M, Wan M, Quintero R, Hobbins JC, Mitchell MD. Prostaglandin concentrations in amniotic fluid of women with intra-amniotic infection and preterm labour. Am J Obstet Gynecol 1987a;157:1461-7.

Romero R, Quintero R, Emamian M, Wan M, Grzyboski C, Hobins JC, Mitchell MD. Arachidonate lipoxygenase metabolites in amniotic fluid of women with intra-amniotic infection and preterm labour. Am J Obstet Gynecol 1987b;157:1454-60.

Romero R, Quintero R, Oyarzun E, King Wu Y, Sabo V, Mazor M, Hobbins JC. Intraamniotic infection and the onset of labour in preterm premature rupture of the membranes. Am J Obstet Gynecol 1988a;159:661-6.

Romero R, Wu YK, Mazor M, Hobbins JC, Mitchell MD. Amniotic fluid 5-Hydroxyeicosatetraenoic acid in preterm labour. Prostaglandins 1988b;36:180-9.

Romero R, Wu YK, Mazor M, Hobbins JC, Mitchell MD. Increased amniotic fluid leukotriene C4 concentration in term human parturition. Am J Obstet Gynecol. 1988c;159:655-7.

Romero R, Hobbins JC, Mitchell MD. Endotoxin stimulates prostaglandin E2 production by human amnion. Obstet Gynecol 1988d;71:227-8.

Romero R, Wu YK, Sirtori M, Oyarzun E, Mazor M, Hobbins JC, Mitchell MD. Amniotic fluid concentrations of prostaglandin F2a, 13,14-dihydro-15-keto-prostaglandin F2a (PGFM) and 11-deoxy-13,14-dihydro-15-keto-11, 16-cyclo-prostaglandin E2 (PGEM-II) in preterm labour. Prostaglandins 1989a;37:149-61.

Romero R, Manogue KR, Mitchell MD, Wu YK, Oyarzun E, Hobbins JC, Cerami A. Cachectin-tumor necrosis factor in the amniotic fluid of women with intraamniotic infection and preterm labour. Am J Obstet Gynecol 1989b;161: 336-41.

Romero R, Brody DT, Oyarzun E, Mazor M, King Wu Y, Hobbins JC, Durum SK. Interleukin-1: A signal for the onset of parturition. Am J Obstet Gynecol 1989c;160:1117-23.

Romero R, Shamma F, Avila C, Jimenez C, Callahan R, Nores J, Mazor M, Brekus CA, Hobbins JC. Infection and labour.VI. Prevalence, microbiology and clinical significance of intramniotic infection in twin gestations with preterm labour. Am J Obstet Gynecol 1990;163:757-61.

Romero R, Quintero R, Nores J, Avila C, Mazor M, Hanaoka S, Hagay Z, Merchant L, Hobbins JC. Amniotic fluid white blood cell count: A rapid and simple test to diagnose microbial invasion of the amniotic cavity and predict preterm delivery. Am J Obstet Gynecol 1991a;165:821-30.

Romero R, Ceska M, Avila C, Mazor M, Behnke E, Lindley I. Neutrophil attractant/activating peptide-1/interleukin-8 in term and preterm parturition. Am J Obstet Gynecol 1991b;165:813-20.

Romero R, Mazor M, Sepulveda W, Avila C, Copeland D, Williams J. Tumor necrosis factor in preterm and term labour. Am J Obstet Gynecol 1992a;166:1576-87.

Romero R, Avila C, Edwin SS, Mitchell MD. Endothelin-1,2 levels are increased in the amniotic fluid of women with preterm labour and microbial invasion of the amniotic cavity. Am J Obstet Gynecol 1992b;166:95-9.

Romero R, Yoon BH, Mazor M, Gomez R, Gonzalez R, Diamond MP, Baumann P, Araneda H, Kenney JS, Cotton DB, Sehgal P. A comparitive study of the diagnostic performance of amniotic fluid glucose, white blood cell count, interleukin-6, and Gram stain in the detection of microbial invasion in patients with premature rupture of membranes. Am J Obstet Gynecol 1993;169:839-51.

Rouquet Y, Paul G, Philippon A, Tournaire M, Nevot P, Chavinie J. The bacteriostatic and bactericidal effect of amniotic fluid. J Gynecol Obstet Biol Reprod Paris 1981;10:119-25.

Roussis P, Rosemond RL, Glass C, Boehm FH. Preterm premature rupture of membranes: Detection of infection. Am J Obstet Gynecol 1991;165:1099-104.

Sachs BP, Stern CM. Activity and characterisation of a low molecular fraction present in human amniotic fluid with broad spectrum antibacterial activity. Br J Obstet Gynaecol 1979 Feb;86;2:81-6.

Saltzman WM, Radomsky ML, Whaley KJ, Cone RA. Antibody diffusion in human cervical mucus. Biophs J 1994 Feb;66:508-15.

Sbarra AJ, Thomas GB, Cetrulo CL, Shakr C, Chaudhury A, Paul B. Effect of bacterial growth on the bursting pressure of fetal membranes in vitro. Obstet Gynecol 1987;70:107-10.

Scane TMN, Hawkins DF. Antibacterial activity in human amniotic fluid:relationship to zinc and phosphate. Br J Obstet Gynaecol. 1984;91:342-8.

Scane TMN, Hawkins DF. Antibacterial activity in human amniotic fluid:dependence on divalent cations. Br J Obstet Gynaecol 1986;93:577-81.

Schlievert P, Johnson W, Galask RP. Bacterial growth inhibition by amniotic fluid VI. Evidence for a zinc-peptide antibacterial system. Am J Obstet Gynecol 1976;125:906-10.

Schlievert P, Johnson W, Galask RP. Bacterial growth inhibition by amniotic fluid VII. The effect of zinc supplementation on bacterial inhibitory activity of amniotic fluids from gestation of 20 weeks. Am J Obstet Gynecol 1977;127: 603-8.

Schlievert P, Johnson W, Galask RP. Isolation of a low molecular weight antibacterial system from human amniotic fluid. Infect Immun 1976;14:1156-66.

Schlievert P, Larsen B, Johnson W, Galask RP. Bacterial growth inhibition by amniotic fluid IV. Studies on the nature of bacterial inhibition with the use of plate count determinations. Am J Obstet Gynecol 1975;122:814-19.

Schmidt W, Klima G. Experimental and histological studies on fetal membrane tensitility and membrane rupture. Zentrabl Gynakol 1989;111:129-41.

Schoonmaker JN, Lawellin DW, Lunt B, McGregor JA. Bacteria and inflammatory cells reduce chorioamniotic membrane integrity and tensile strength. Obstet Gynecol 1989;74:590-5.

Seo K, McGregor JA, French JI. Preterm birth is associated with increased risk of maternal and neonatal infection. Obstet Gynecol 1992;79:75-80.

Sherman MP, Chance KH, Goetzman BW. Grams stain of tracheal secretions predict neonatal bacteraemia. Am J Dis Child 1984;138:848-50.

Siegel JD, McCracken GH. Sepsis neonatorum. NEJM 1981;304:642-7.

Silver HM, Sperling RS, StClair PJ, Gibbs RS. Evidence relating bacterial vaginosis to intramniotic infection. Am J Obstet Gynecol 1989;161:808-12.

Skinner SJM, Campos GA, Liggins GC. Collagen content of human amniotic membranes: effect of gestation length and premature rupture. Obstet Gynecol1981;57:487-489.

Skoll MA, Moretti ML, Sibai BM. The incidence of positive amniotic fluid cultures in patients in preterm labour with intact membranes. Am J Obstet Gynecol 1989;161:813-16.

Squire E, Favara B, Todd J. Diagnosis of neonatal bacterial infection: Hematologic and pathologic findings in fatal and non fatal cases. Pediatrics 1979;64:60-4.

Stefanovic I, Stefanovic J, Bucova M, Murgasova I, Sasko A. Antiphagocytic activity of human amniotic fluid. Bratisl Lek Listy 1993;94:293-6.

Sugarman B, Agbor P. The binding of chlamydia trachomatis and zinc to McCoy cells. Infection 1987;15:35-9.

Sugarman B. Zinc and Infection. Rev Infect Dis 1983;1:137-47.

Svensson L, Ingemarsson I, Mardh P. chorioamnionitis and the isolation of microorganisms from the placenta. Obstet Gynecol 1986;67:403-9.

Taylor J, Garite TJ. Premature rupture of membranes before fetal viability. Obstet Gynecol 1984;64:615-20.

Thibeault DW, Emmanouilides GC. Prolonged rupture of fetal membranes and decreased frequency of respiratory distress syndrome and patent ductus arteriosus in preterm infants. Am J Obstet Gynecol 1977;129:43-6.

Thilaganathan B, Carroll SG, Plachouras N, Makrydimas G, Nicolaides KH. Fetal immunological and haematological changes in intrauterine infection. Br J Obstet Gynaecol 1994;101:418-21.

Thompson PJ, Greenough A, Gamsu HR, Nicolaides KH, Philpott-Howard J. Congenital bacterial sepsis in very preterm infants. J Med Microbiol 1992;36: 1-4.

Thompson PJ, Greenough A, Hird MF, Philpott-Howard J, Gamsu HR. Nosocomial bacterial infections in very low birth weight infants. Eur J Ped 1992;151:451-4.

Towers CV, Lewis DF, Asrat T, Gardner K, Perlow JH. The effect of colonization with group B streptococci on the latency phase of patients with preterm PROM. Am J Obstet Gynecol 1993;169:1139-43.

Trautman MS, Dudley DJ, Edwin SS, Collmer D, Mitchell MD. Amnion cell biosynthesis of interleukin-8:regulation by inflammatory cytokines. J Cell Physiol 1992;153:38-43.

Vadillo-Ortega F, Gonzalez-Avila G, Karchmer S, Cruz NM, Ayala-Ruiz A, Lama MS. Collagen metabolism in premature rupture of amniotic membranes. Obstet Gynecol 1990;75:84-7.

Vadillo-Ortega F, Gonzalez-Avila G, Villaneuva-Diaz C, Banales JL, Selman-Lama M, Duran AA. Human amniotic fluid modulation of collagenase production in cultured fibroblasts. Am J Obstet Gynecol 1991;164:664-8.

Vintzileos AM, Campbell WA, Nochimson DJ, Weinbaum PJ, Escoto DT, Mirochnick MH. Qualitative amniotic fluid volume versus amniocentesis in predicting infection in preterm premature rupture of the membranes. Obstet Gynecol 1986;67:579-83.

Visser VE, Hall RT. Lumbar puncture in the evaluation of suspected neonatal sepsis. J Pediatr 1980;96:1063-7.

Visser VE, Hall RT. Urine culture in the evaluation of suspected neonatal sepsis. J Pediatr 1979;94:635-8.

Volochine B, Cazabat AM, Chretien FC, Kuntsmann JM. Structure of human cervical mucus from light scattering measurements. Hum Reprod 1988;3: 577-82.

Wahbeh CJ, Hill GB, Eden RD, Gall SA. Intra-amniotic bacterial colonization in premature labour. Am J Obstet Gynecol 1984;148:739-43.

Walsh SW. 5 hydroxyeicososatetraenoic acid, leukotriene C4 and prostaglandin F2 alpha in amniotic fluid before and during term and preterm labour. Am J Obstet Gynecol 1989;161:1352-60.

Watts DH, Krohn MA, Hillier SL, Escenbach DA. The association of occult amniotic fluid infection with gestational age and neonatal outcome among women in preterm labour. Obstet Gynecol 1992;79:351-7.

Wilson JC, Levy DL, Preston LW. Premature rupture of membranes prior to term: Consequences of nonintervention. Obstet Gynecol 1982;60:601-6.

Zlatnik FJ, Gellhaus TM, Benda JA, Koontz FP, Burmeister LF. Histologic chorioamnionitis, microbial infection and prematurity. Obstet Gynecol 1990;76:355-9.

Zuckerman H, Reiss V, Rubenstein I. Inhibition of human preterm labour by indomethacin. Obstet Gynecol 1974;44:787-92.

Preterm prelabour amniorrhexis: detection of infection

OVERVIEW

AMNIOCENTESIS AND CORDOCENTESIS
- Gram stain
- Leukocyte count
- Glucose
- Other tests on amniotic fluid
- Fetal haematological indices

MATERNAL ASSESSMENT
- Clinical signs, leukocyte count and C-reactive protein
- Lower genital tract swabs

FETAL ASSESSMENT
- Fetal activity
- Amniotic fluid volume
- Doppler studies of the placental and fetal circulation
- Fetal blood gases

CONCLUSIONS

OVERVIEW

In pregnancies complicated by preterm prelabour amniorrhexis, there is a risk of intrauterine infection which is associated with maternal and perinatal mortality and morbidity. In the clinical management of pregnancies with amniorrhexis, it is aimed to distinguish those without infection, that can be managed expectantly, from those with infection where early delivery and/or antibiotic therapy can be undertaken.

The diagnosis of microbial invasion of the amniotic cavity and fetal bacteraemia can be made by culture of amniotic fluid and fetal blood obtained by amniocentesis and cordocentesis (see Chapter 2). However, the delay in obtaining results from these cultures has stimulated the search for rapid tests such as the Gram stain in amniotic fluid and leukocyte count in fetal blood.

Several studies have attempted to predict intrauterine infection non-invasively by assessment of (i) maternal heart rate, temperature, leukocyte count and serum C-reactive protein concentration, (ii) cultures of lower genital tract swabs, and (iii) fetal assessment by Doppler studies of the placental and fetal circulation, fetal activity, fetal heart rate patterns and amniotic fluid volume.

AMNIOCENTESIS AND CORDOCENTESIS

The diagnosis of intrauterine infection is made by culture of amniotic fluid and fetal blood. However, it takes at least two days before the results of culture are available and consequently, a series of rapid tests has been developed to predict the presence of infection. This is particularly important since, in the presence of fetal bacteraemia, spontaneous delivery occurs within a few days of amniorrhexis and the results of culture may not be ready in time for purposeful obstetric intervention.

Gram stain

Bacteria are stained with methyl violet and iodine; they are then washed with alcohol and counterstained with a dye of a different colour. Gram positive organisms retain the original stain and appear violet while Gram negative organisms are decolorised by alcohol and are stained pink by the counterstain.

In pregnancies with preterm prelabour amniorrhexis, a positive amniotic fluid Gram stain has a high sensitivity (60-80%) and an acceptably low false positive rate (3-5%) in the prediction of intrauterine infection with aerobic or anaerobic organisms. However, the Gram stain does not identify *Mycoplasma* species and, when these organisms are included, the sensitivity of the test is only 24-50% (Table 3.1).

Table 3.1. True positive rate (TP) and false positive rate (FP) for amniotic fluid Gram stain in the prediction of positive amniotic fluid cultures in preterm prelabour amniorrhexis. In all studies the fluid was cultured for aerobic and anaerobic organisms, but in some *Mycoplasma* species (Uu/Mh) were also looked for.

Author	N	Uu/Mh	TP	FP
Garite & Freeman 1982	86	No	70%	3%
Cotton *et al* 1984	41	No	83%	3%
Broekhuizen *et al* 1985	53	No	60%	5%
Carroll *et al* 1995a	80	No	80%	3%
Vintzileos *et al* 1986a	79	Yes	34%	0%
Coultrip *et al* 1992	29	Yes	50%	18
Romero *et al* 1993	110	Yes	24%	1%
Carroll *et al* 1995a	80	Yes	40%	4%

Leukocyte count

Intrauterine infection, with aerobic and anaerobic organisms as well as with *Mycoplasma* species, is associated with increased amniotic fluid leukocyte count (Figure 3.1, Carroll *et al* 1995a). However, in contrast to the Gram stain, amniotic fluid leukocyte count does not provide clinically useful information on intrauterine infection because, for acceptably low false positive rates (<5%), the sensitivity of the test in the prediction of infection is less than 25% (Table 3.2).

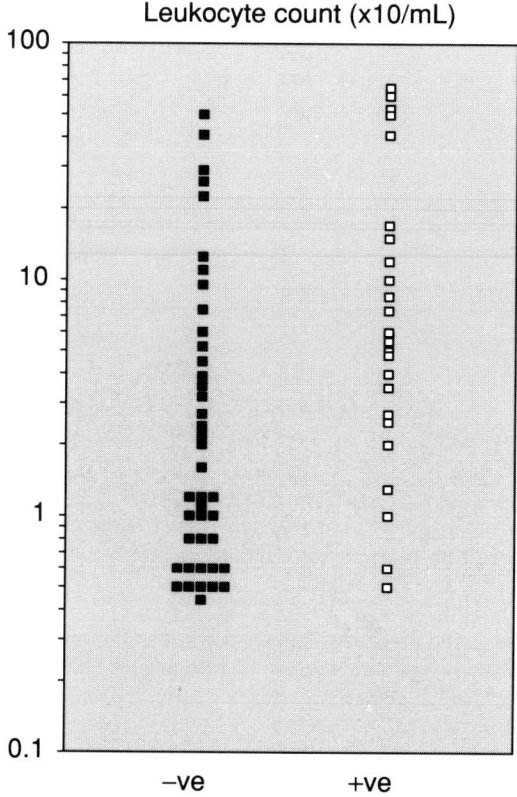

Figure 3.1. Values of amniotic fluid leukocyte count (LCx10/mm³) in patients with positive (□) and negative (■) amniotic fluid cultures (Carroll *et al* 1995a).

Table 3.2. True positive rate (TP) and false positive rate (FP) for different cut-off levels of leukocyte count (LC) in amniotic fluid in the prediction of positive amniotic fluid cultures in preterm prelabour amniorrhexis. In all studies the fluid was cultured for aerobic and anaerobic organisms, but in some *Mycoplasma* species (Uu/Mh) were also looked for.

Author	Leukocytes	N	Uu/Mh	TP	FP
Garite *et al* 1979	>1/HPF	30	No	22%	5%
Garite & Freeman 1982	Present	86	No	15%	15%
Coultrip *et al* 1992	>6/OIF	29	Yes	16%	-
Romero *et al* 1993	>30/mm³	110	No	57%	20%
Carroll *et al* 1995a	LC≥500/mm³	67	Yes	17%	0%
	LC≥500/mm³	67	No	17%	4%
	LC>30/mm³	67	Yes	66%	35%
	LC>30/mm³	67	No	75%	40%

HPF = high power field, OIF = oil immersion field.

Glucose

In normal pregnancy the amniotic fluid concentration of glucose decreases with gestation from a mean of 46 mg/dL at 16 weeks to 16 mg/dL at term (Weiss *et al* 1985). In the presence of infection the amniotic fluid concentration of glucose is often reduced because many organisms use glucose as a substrate (Table 3.3). However, the sensitivity of this test is low because glucose metabolism may be organism dependent. For example, *Mycoplasma* species do not use glucose as a substrate (Klein 1990).

Table 3.3. True positive rate (TP) and false positive rate (FP) for amniotic fluid glucose concentration in the prediction of positive amniotic fluid cultures in preterm prelabour amniorrhexis.

Author	Glucose	N	TP	FP
Gauthier *et al* 1991	< 16 mg/dL	91	49%	2%
Coultrip *et al* 1992	< 10 mg/dL	29	25%	36%
	< 15 mg/dL	29	33%	42%
Romero *et al* 1993	< 10 mg/dL	110	57%	26%
	< 14 mg/dL	110	71%	49%

Other tests on amniotic fluid

Limulus amoebocyte lysate assay

This is a rapid bioassay for endotoxin on the cell wall of Gram negative organisms and is based on the gelation of the lysate of blood cells (amoebocytes) of the horseshoe crab, *Limulus polyphemus* (Elin & Hosseini 1985). The assay is performed by adding amniotic fluid to *Limulus* amoebocyte lysate and incubating the mixture for one hour. A positive test result is scored when a solid adherent gel is present on inversion of the tube. Since endotoxin is present only in Gram negative bacteria, false negative results occur with infections caused by Gram positive bacteria, *Mycoplasma* species and fungi (Table 3.4).

Leukocyte esterase activity

This is a product of polymorphonuclear leukocytes and, in the presence of intra-amniotic infection, the activity of the enzyme is increased; this is detected by the change in colour of a test strip within a few minutes after the addition of amniotic fluid (Kusimi *et al* 1981). Three studies evaluating this test in pregnancies with preterm prelabour amniorrhexis have reported conflicting results (Table 3.4).

Table 3.4. True positive rate (TP) and false positive rate (FP) for various tests performed on amniotic fluid in the prediction of positive amniotic fluid cultures in preterm prelabour amniorrhexis.

Author	Test	N	TP	FP
Coultrip *et al* 1992	*Limulus* amoebocyte lysate	29	25%	6%
Romero *et al* 1987	*Limulus* amoebocyte lysate	65	69%	5%
Coultrip *et al* 1992	Leukocyte esterase	29	25%	59%
Romero *et al* 1988a	Leukocyte esterase	171	19%	13%
Fisk 1987	Leukocyte esterase	20	83%	14%
Romero *et al* 1988b	Gas-liquid chromatography	26	68%	57%
Robert *et al* 1988	Fibronectin $\leq$ 20 µg/mL	30	27%	27%
Robert *et al* 1988	Fibronectin $\leq$ 40 µg/mL	30	87%	93%
O'Brien *et al* 1990	α_1-Antitrypsin<30 mg/dL	70	31%	77%

Gas-liquid chromatography

Bacteria produce metabolites such as volatile fatty and non-volatile organic acids that can be detected in amniotic fluid by gas-liquid chromatography.

Gravett *et al* (1982) reported a 93% sensitivity of this test in the prediction of positive amniotic fluid cultures in pregnancies with preterm prelabour amniorrhexis and preterm labour with intact membranes; the false positive rate was 9%. However, a study in pregnancies with preterm prelabour amniorrhexis reported that the respective true and false positive rates of the test were 68% and 57% (Table 3.4).

Fibronectins

These are a family of high molecular weight glycoproteins which act as non-specific opsonins that promote phagocytosis of bacteria by macrophages (Hill *et al* 1984, Van De Water 1985).

Fibronectins have been identified in the amniotic fluid of normal pregnancies (Hess *et al* 1986) and it was hypothesised that intrauterine infection may be the consequence of deficiency in amniotic fluid concentration of these substances (Robert *et al* 1988). However, the amniotic fluid concentration of fibronectins in pregnancies with preterm prelabour amniorrhexis and positive amniotic fluid cultures was not significantly different from those with negative cultures (Table 3.4).

α_1-Antitrypsin

Granulocyte elastase, released from inflammatory cells in the fetal membranes, utilises α_1-antitrypsin as a substrate and it was therefore suggested that the amniotic fluid concentration of the latter may be reduced in the presence of infection. However, the amniotic fluid concentration of α_1-antitrypsin in pregnancies with preterm prelabour amniorrhexis and positive amniotic fluid cultures was not significantly different from those with negative cultures (Table 3.4).

Cytokines

The primary aim for the study of these substances has been the better understanding of the pathophysiology of preterm prelabour amniorrhexis and infection, and the interrelation between infection and preterm labour (see Chapter 2; Table 3.5). However, alterations in the amniotic fluid concentration of these substances in the presence of infection can potentially be utilised for the development of rapid tests to aid clinical management.

Table 3.5. True positive rate (TP) and false positive rate (FP) for amniotic fluid concentration of cytokines in the prediction of positive amniotic fluid cultures in preterm prelabour amniorrhexis.

Author	Cytokine	N	TP	FP
Romero *et al* 1989	Interleukin-1β (>10 IU/mL)	66	59%	11%
Romero *et al* 1992	Tumour necrosis factor (>60 g/mL)	72	48%	2%
Romero *et al* 1993	Interleukin-6 (>7.9 ng/mL)	110	81%	25%

Fetal haematological indices

In normal fetuses, the lymphocyte count increases linearly with gestation and at 20 weeks the levels are approximately 50% of those at term (Davies *et al* 1992). The relatively high numbers of lymphocytes from early pregnancy may be reconciled with the need to acquire immunological tolerance and antigen recognition functions. The latter may be essential in combating viral infections which can cross the placenta.

Neutrophil counts are very low (approximately 10% of those at term) until 32 weeks and increase exponentially thereafter to reach adult levels at term. Presumably, in evolutionary terms, the placenta acts as an effective barrier to most bacteria, and therefore the acquisition of host defence mechanisms directed against bacterial infection is only necessary in the third trimester in preparation for extrauterine life.

Fetal blood sampling by cordocentesis in pregnancies with preterm prelabour amniorrhexis has demonstrated fetal leukocytosis and neutrophilia which were most marked in bacteraemic fetuses (Carroll *et al* 1995b, Figure 3.2). In contrast, the lymphocyte count, haemoglobin concentration and platelet count are normal (Figure 3.3).

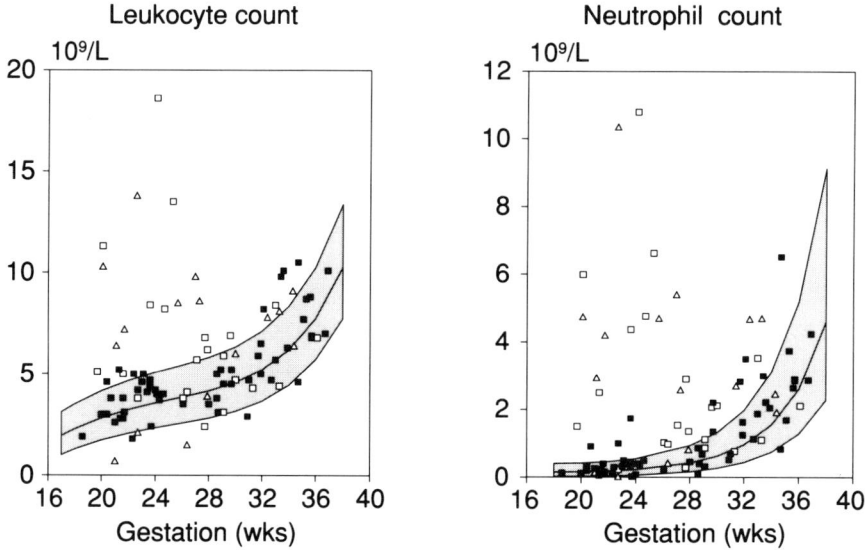

Figure 3.2. Fetal leukocyte and neutrophil counts in patients with preterm prelabour amniorrhexis plotted on the appropriate normal range for gestation (shaded area, mean ± 2 SDs). (■)= patients with negative fetal blood and amniotic fluid cultures, (□)= patients with positive amniotic fluid and negative fetal blood cultures, (Δ)= patients with positive fetal blood cultures. Adapted from Carroll *et al* 1995b.

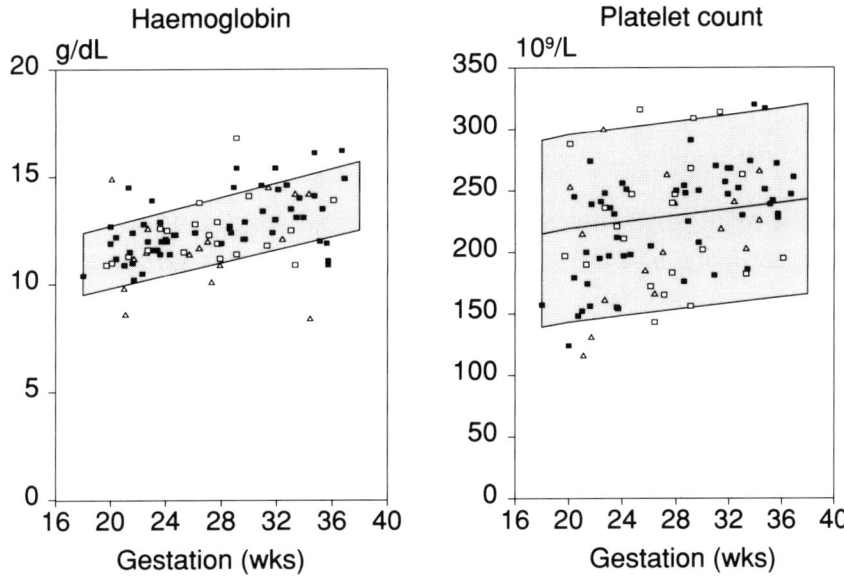

Figure 3.3. Fetal haemoglobin concentration and platelet count in patients with preterm prelabour amniorrhexis plotted on the appropriate normal range for gestation (shaded area, mean ± 2 SDs). (■)= patients with negative fetal blood and amniotic fluid cultures, (□)= patients with positive amniotic fluid and negative fetal blood cultures, (△)= patients with positive fetal blood cultures. Adapted from Carroll *et al* 1995b.

The findings that fetal bacteraemia is associated with leukocytosis and neutrophilia are in apparent contradiction with the well described association between neonatal sepsis and neutropenia (Christensen & Rothstein 1980a; Gerdes 1991).

It is possible that intrauterine infection causes mobilisation of neutrophils and therefore fetal neutrophilia. Ultimately the neutrophil storage pool is exhausted (Christensen & Rothstein 1980a, Christensen *et al* 1982) and the neonates are neutropenic. In this respect, the fetus may not be dissimilar to the adult where infection is associated with neutrophilia, but when the infection is overwhelming there is neutropenia.

Fetal leukocytosis is also present in cases of microbial invasion of the amniotic fluid in the absence of fetal bacteraemia. In these cases, fetal leukocytosis may occur in response to localised infection in the chorionic villi or in the lung. Animal studies have demonstrated that, in the neonate, neutrophil mobilisation from the storage pool is more sensitive to localised stimuli than in the adult (Christensen & Rothstein 1980b), and this exaggerated response may also occur in utero.

The mean fetal leukocyte and neutrophil counts in the group with negative fetal blood and amniotic fluid cultures were also significantly higher than normal but not as high as in the infected groups. The most likely cause for the fetal leukocytosis in these cases is the stress associated with amniorrhexis; previous studies have reported increased amniotic fluid concentrations of cortisol and cytokines in amniorrhexis without infection (Gewolb *et al* 1977, Potter *et al* 1992).

MATERNAL ASSESSMENT

Clinical signs, leukocyte count and C-reactive protein

The cardinal signs of infection that constitute the cornerstones of clinical monitoring are maternal tachycardia, pyrexia and leukocytosis. In addition, measurement of maternal C-reactive protein, an acute-phase protein produced by hepatocytes in response to inflammation or infection, has been proposed as a sensitive index of intrauterine infection.

The studies examining the value of these parameters in the prediction of intrauterine infection in pregnancies complicated by preterm prelabour amniorrhexis have reported a wide range of true positive and false positive rates (Table 3.6).

The most likely explanation for the disparities in results from the various studies are the different end-points used for the diagnosis of infection, which included clinical or histological evidence of chorioamnionitis, positive amniotic fluid and/or fetal blood culture.

Clinical chorioamnionitis

As shown in Table 3.7, there were major differences between the various studies in the criteria used for the diagnosis of clinical chorioamnionitis.

Table 3.6. True positive rate (TP) and false positive rate (FP) of maternal pyrexia (temperature at least 38°C), leukocytosis (leukocyte count above 12.5x10^9/L or 16x10^9/L or 20x10^9/L or more than 30% above basal levels) and raised C-reactive protein (above 1.2 mg/dL or 1.5 mg/dL or 2 mg/dL) in the prediction of intrauterine infection. The diagnosis of infection included the presence of clinical signs (see Table 3.7), histological evidence of chorioamnionitis, positive amniotic fluid cultures (+ve AFC), or a combination of the three (Mixed).

Author	Parameter	N	Infection	TP	FP
Garite & Freeman 1982	T≥38°C	86	+ve AFC	55%	8%
Broekhuizen *et al* 1985	T≥38°C	53	+ve AFC	20%	0%
Ismail *et al* 1985	T≥38°C	100	Histological	17%	3%
Ismail *et al* 1985	T≥38°C	100	Clinical	56%	2%
Garite & Freeman 1982	LC>20x10^9/L	247	Clinical	6%	5%
Garite & Freeman 1982	LC>10x10^9/L	247	Clinical	83%	67%
Hawrylyshyn *et al* 1983	LC>12.5x10^9/L	52	Histological	80%	38%
Ismail *et al* 1985	LC>30%basal	100	Histological	23%	14%
Ismail *et al* 1985	LC>30%basal	100	Clinical	47%	15%
Romem & Artal 1984	LC>12.5x10^9/L	51	Clinical	43%	18%
Romem & Artal 1984	LC>16x10^9/L	51	Clinical	29%	5%
Hawrylyshyn *et al* 1983	CRP>1.2mg/dL	52	Histological	88%	4%
Farb *et al* 1983	CRP>2mg/dL	24	Histological	80%	32%
Ismail *et al* 1985	CRP>2mg/dL	100	Histological	67%	19%
Kornman *et al* 1988	CRP>1.2mg/dL	63	Histological	73%	30%
Farb *et al* 1983	CRP>2mg/dL	31	Clinical	55%	27%
Romem & Artal 1984	CRP>2mg/dL	51	Clinical	86%	14%
Ismail *et al* 1985	CRP>2mg/dL	100	Clinical	82%	45%
Ernest *et al* 1987	CRP>2mg/dL	85	Mixed	60%	36%
Evans *et al* 1980	CRP>2mg/dL	36	Mixed	80%	0%
Watts *et al* 1993	CRP>1.5mg/dL	82	Clinical	79%	49%
Watts *et al* 1993	CRP>1.5mg/dL	82	Histological	46%	62%
Watts *et al* 1993	CRP>1.5mg/dL	82	+ve AFC	100%	24%

In some studies a mixture of criteria was used. For example, Ernest *et al* (1987) defined infection by either the presence of clinical signs (see Table 3.7), or positive amniotic fluid culture, or the presence of pathogens isolated from the placenta at the time of caesarean section. Similarly, Evans *et al* (1980) defined infection by either the presence of clinical signs (see Table 3.7), or the presence of histological chorioamnionitis, or positive neonatal blood culture.

Table 3.7. Criteria for the diagnosis of clinical chorioamnionitis used in different studies.

Feature	1	2	3	4	5	6	7	8	9
Maternal pyrexia	*	*	*	*	*	*	*	*	*
Maternal tachycardia						*	*	*	
Maternal leukocytosis		*		*		*		*	*
Uterine tenderness				*	*	*	*	*	*
Offensive vaginal discharge			*			*	*	*	
Fetal tachycardia			*			*	*	*	*

1: Pyrexia of no other obvious cause (Garite & Freeman 1982, Romem & Artal 1984)
2: Any one of the two features (Ismail *et al* 1985)
3 Any one of the three features (Evans *et al* 1980)
4: Any one of the three features (Ferguson *et al* 1985)
5: Both features (Miller *et al* 1990)
6: Any two of the six features (Vintzileos *et al* 1986a, Roussis *et al* 1991)
7: Pyrexia and one of the other four features (Del Valle *et al* 1992)
8: Pyrexia and two of the other five features (Ernest *et al* 1987, Watts *et al* 1993)
9: Pyrexia or leukocytosis and uterine tenderness or fetal tachycardia (Farb *et al* 1983)

Since clinical chorioamnionitis may be a late manifestation of infection, those studies examining patients with clinical signs have inevitably reported the highest incidences of pyrexia and leukocytosis. Indeed in one study the parameter under investigation was included in the criteria for the diagnosis of infection (Ismail *et al* 1985). In another study, that reported a high incidence of maternal pyrexia in the presence of positive amniotic fluid cultures, temperatures were recorded even 19 days after the amniocentesis (Garite & Freeman 1982)

Histological chorioamnionitis

The diagnosis of histological chorioamnionitis is based on the demonstration of polymorphonuclear leukocyte infiltration of the intervillous space below the chorionic plate, the amniotic membranes or umbilical cord vessels.

The degree of inflammation may be graded according to: (i) the site of inflammation (Perkins *et al* 1987), into funisitis (umbilical cord and Whartons jelly), or chorioamnionitis (membranes and chorionic plate), (ii) the number of polymorphs seen per high power field on microscopic examination (Guzick & Winn 1985, Perkins *et al* 1987), into significant (more than four cells) or sparse (less than four cells), (iii) the depth to which polymorphs have infiltrated the amnion and chorion (Mueller-Heubach *et al* 1990), into mild (neutrophils present in the subchorionic space) through to severe (dense infiltration of neutrophils extending from the subchorionic space throughout the chorion).

The use of histological chorioamnionitis as an end-point for intrauterine infection may be inappropriate. Studies examining the relation between histological chorioamnionitis and cultures of placental swabs have demonstrated that (i) about one third of placentae with histological chorioamnionitis are culture negative, and (ii) about one third of infected membranes are free of inflammation (Table 3.8).

Table 3.8. Studies examining the relation between histological chorioamnionitis and the results of placental cultures.

Author	N	Histology positive Culture negative	Histology negative Culture positive
Pankuch *et al* 1984	64	28%	15%
Svensson *et al* 1986	79	30%	45%
Quinn *et al* 1987	43	29%	28%
Hillier *et al* 1988	94	28%	22%
Zlatnick *et al* 1990	95	27%	27%
Total	**375**	**28%**	**29%**

Since histological chorioamnionitis is both an insensitive and non-specific marker of intrauterine infection, it is not surprising that, in the preterm prelabour amniorrhexis studies that examined maternal pyrexia, leukocytosis or increased C-reactive protein in relation to histological chorioamnionitis, the false positive rate varied from 3% to 62% (Table 3.6).

Another factor that may have contributed to the high sensitivity and high false positive rate of leukocytosis in the prediction of chorioamnionitis in some studies is the administration of corticosteroids to the patients (Hawrylyshyn *et al* 1983); steroids are known to cause an increase in the polymorphonuclear leukocyte count.

Positive amniotic fluid or fetal blood cultures

Carroll *et al* (1995c) diagnosed intrauterine infection if the cultures of fetal blood and/or amniotic fluid, obtained by cordocentesis and amniocentesis, were positive. They reported that maternal heart rate, temperature, leukocyte count and C-reactive protein did not provide sensitive prediction of infection irrespective of whether this was defined by positive amniotic fluid or positive fetal blood cultures (Table 3.9; Figures 3.4 and 3.5).

The most likely explanation for the low sensitivity of the various maternal tests in the prediction of positive amniotic fluid cultures in this study, compared to previous ones, is that Carroll *et al* (1995c) examined *Mycoplasma* species in addition to aerobic and anaerobic organisms.

Mycoplasma species are less likely than other bacterial infections to produce clinical signs (Cassell *et al* 1986). However, these organisms are important because they cause neonatal pneumonia and meningitis and recent evidence indicates that *Ureaplasma*

Table 3.9. Incidence of maternal pyrexia, tachycardia, leukocytosis and high C-reactive protein in 75 pregnancies with preterm prelabour amniorrhexis. In this study amniocentesis and cordocentesis were performed and the diagnosis of intrauterine infection was made on the basis of positive amniotic fluid and/or fetal blood cultures (Carroll *et al* 1995c).

Parameter	Amniotic fluid		Fetal blood	
	+ve	- ve	+ ve	- ve
Pyrexia (>38°C)	7%	0%	16%	0%
Tachycardia ($\geq$100 bpm)	14%	2%	25%	3%
Leukocytosis ($\geq$15 x10^9/L)	14%	6%	16%	8%
C-reactive protein (>2mg/dL)	28%	15%	33%	17%

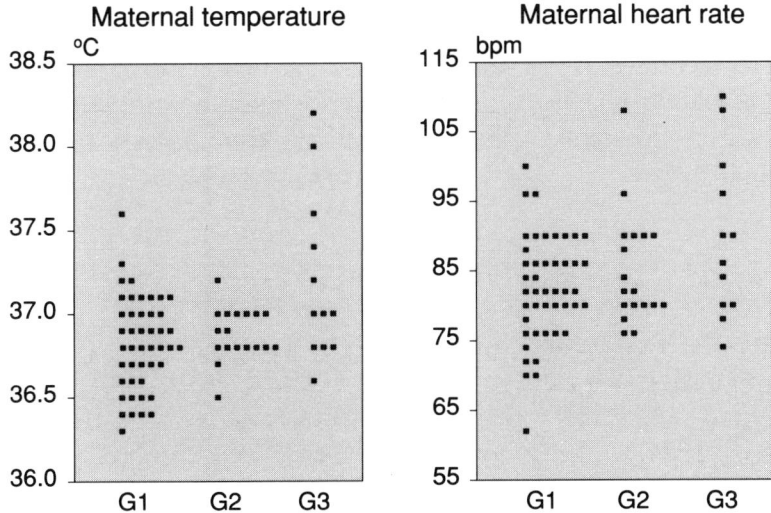

Figure 3.4. Maternal temperature and heart rate in pregnancies with preterm prelabour amniorrhexis. The diagnosis of intrauterine infection was made on the basis of positive amniotic fluid and/or fetal blood cultures (Carroll *et al* 1995c). In group 1 (G1) amniotic fluid and fetal blood cultures were negative, in group 2 (G2) amniotic fluid cultures were positive and in group 3 (G3) fetal blood cultures were positive.

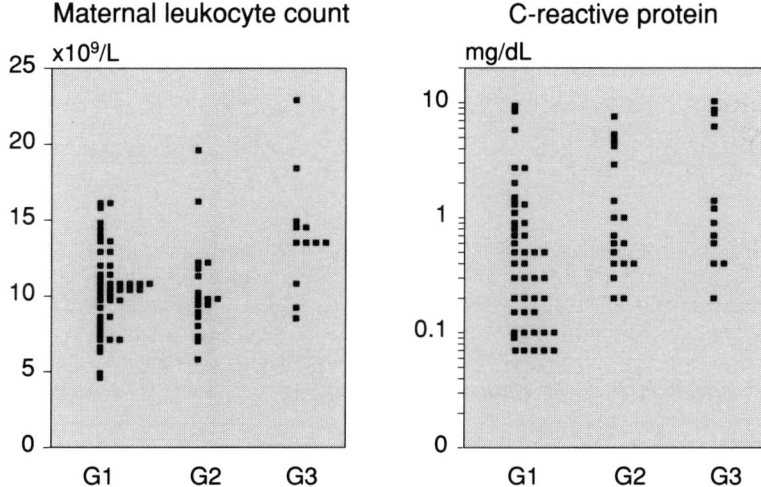

Figure 3.5. Maternal leukocyte count and C-reactive protein in pregnancies with preterm prelabour amniorrhexis. The diagnosis of intrauterine infection was made on the basis of positive amniotic fluid and/or fetal blood cultures (Carroll *et al* 1995c). In group 1 (G1) amniotic fluid and fetal blood cultures were negative, in group 2 (G2) amniotic fluid cultures were positive and in group 3 (G3) fetal blood cultures were positive.

urealyticum is the commonest organism isolated from the central nervous system and lower respiratory tract of premature neonates (Wientzen 1990, Cassell *et al* 1993).

Lower genital tract swabs

Intrauterine infection from organisms found in the lower genital tract has been implicated in both the aetiology and adverse sequelae of preterm prelabour amniorrhexis (see Chapter 2). Consequently, an essential part of the clinical management of such pregnancies is culture of swabs from the vagina or endocervix. However, there is a sparsity of studies that evaluate such cultures in the prediction of intrauterine infection.

Recently, Carroll *et al* (1995d) examined the relation of genital tract flora to micro-organisms found in fetal blood and amniotic fluid in women with preterm prelabour amniorrhexis (Table 3.10).

Table 3.10. True positive rate (TP) and false positive rate (FP) of positive cultures from the lower genital tract in the prediction of positive amniotic fluid and fetal blood cultures in 97 cases of preterm prelabour amniorrhexis (Carroll *et al* 1995d). For *Mycoplasma* species only amniotic fluid was cultured.

Organism	Amniotic fluid		Fetal blood	
	TP	FP	TP	FP
Aerobes and/or anaerobes	53%	25%	40%	24%
Candida albicans	100%	9%	100%	7%
Streptococcus agalactiae	67%	6%	50%	5%
Other	45%	11%	33%	13%
Mycoplasma species	85%	35%	-	-
Any organism	76%	58%	-	-

In more than 75% of cases with positive amniotic fluid cultures, the same organisms were recovered from vaginal and/or endocervical swabs. This finding is compatible with the hypothesis that the lower genital tract is the source of the offending organisms in intrauterine infection associated with amniorrhexis. However, the incidence of positive cultures from the lower genital tract in the patients with amniorrhexis was similar to that in normal pregnancies (Table 3.11).

Positive genital tract cultures for aerobic and anaerobic organisms predicted 40% of positive fetal blood and 53% of positive amniotic fluid cultures with false positive rates of 24% and 25%, respectively. The true and false positive rates for genital tract colonisation with *Mycoplasma* species in the prediction of amniotic fluid infection with these organisms were 85% and 35%, respectively (Table 3.10).

The incidence of various micro-organisms in the lower genital tract in patients with preterm prelabour amniorrhexis (Carroll *et al* 1995d) was similar to that in previous studies of swabs taken at routine antenatal visits in normal pregnancies. Thus, the incidence of *Mycoplasma* species was 55% in patients with amniorrhexis compared to the mean incidence of 68% in 11 previous studies. Aerobic and/or anaerobic cultures were positive in 23% of the patients with amniorrhexis and in 15% of cases in one previous report on normal pregnancies. *Streptococcus agalactiae* was found in 7% of the cases with amniorrhexis and in 15% (range 3-18%) of cases in nine previous reports (Table 3.11).

Table 3.11. Prevalence of genital tract colonisation with aerobes or anaerobes (A/An), *Streptococcus agalactiae* (Sa*)*, *Ureaplasma urealyticum* (Uu) or *Mycoplasma hominis* (Mh) at routine antenatal visits.

Author	N	A/An	Sa	Uu	Mh
Harrison *et al* 1979	98	?	?	48%	10%
Harrison *et al* 1983	1,365	?	?	72%	23%
Hardy *et al* 1984	115	Present	?	90%	75%
Minkoff *et al* 1984	233	Present	10%	65%	40%
Bobitt *et al* 1985	718	?	6%	?	?
Berman *et al* 1987	1,163	?	?	81%	50%
Sweet *et al* 1987	3,293	?	14%	68%	19%
Alger *et al* 1988	84	?	4%	?	?
McDonald *et al* 1989	692	?	13%	?	?
Vonsee *et al* 1989	698	?	?	24%	5%
McGregor *et al* 1990	229	Present	3%	68%	13%
Carey *et al* 1991	4,934	Present	?	66%	28%
Hillier *et al* 1992	7,918	Present	18%	73%	30%
McDonald *et al* 1992	786	15%	11%	35%	6%
Katz *et al* 1994	1,681	?	14%	?	?
Total	**24,007**		**15%**	**68%**	**27%**

The findings that (i) the incidence of positive cultures from the lower genital tract in women with amniorrhexis is similar to that in normal pregnancies and (ii) cultures from the lower genital tract provide non-specific prediction of intrauterine infection suggest that other factors, apart from mere colonisation of the lower genital tract, are implicated in amniorrhexis and intrauterine infection.

Possible factors include differences in host defence mechanisms, such as antimicrobial properties of amniotic fluid and variation in the inherent strength of amniotic membranes, the number and virulence of different organisms and pathogenicity of different strains of a particular species.

The inability to isolate aerobic and/or anaerobic organisms from the lower genital tract in 47% of the cases with positive amniotic fluid cultures reflects the difficulty of establishing growth of micro-organisms from swabs; failure of bacteria to survive on swabs has been attributed to the low pH of processed cotton-wool and the presence of toxic materials in the wood sticks (Dadd *et al* 1970). An additional and/or alternative explanation is that in some patients the presence of organisms in the lower genital tract is transient (Hillier *et al* 1992).

The incidence of positive amniotic fluid cultures in the study of Carroll *et al* (1995d) was 36%, which is the same as the mean of four previous studies in pregnancies with preterm prelabour amniorrhexis that also examined the amniotic fluid for *Mycoplasma* species in addition to aerobes and anaerobes (Romero *et al* 1988c, Dudley *et al* 1991, Gauthier *et al* 1992, Coultrip & Grossman 1992).

Fetal bacteraemia was found in 33% of the pregnancies with positive amniotic fluid cultures, and in 4% of those with negative cultures (Carroll *et al* 1995d). Possible mechanisms for entry of bacteria into the fetal circulation include transfer across the fetal lungs after aspiration of infected amniotic fluid, or transplacental migration from the decidua basalis into the chorionic villi. Studies examining the relation between positive amniotic fluid cultures and neonatal sepsis in pregnancies with amniorrhexis reported that the incidence of sepsis was about 10% (see Chapter 2).

Table 3.13. Criteria for scoring biophysical variables according to Vintzileos *et al* (1983).

Non-stress test

Fetal heart rate monitoring is carried out for a 20-minute period and a score is given according to the total number of accelerations with an amplitude of at least 15 bpm and a duration of at least 15 seconds.

Score 2: Five or more accelerations
Score 1: Two to four accelerations
Score 0: One or no accelerations

Fetal movements

Ultrasound examination is carried out for a maximum of 30 minutes and a score is given according to the number of episodes of gross (trunk and limbs) fetal movements.

Score 2: At least three episodes of movements
Score 1: One or two episodes of movements
Score 0: No episodes of movements

Fetal breathing movements

Ultrasound examination is carried out for a maximum of 30 minutes and a score is given according to the number of episodes of fetal breathing lasting for at least 30 to 60 seconds.

Score 2: At least one episode of breathing lasting for at least 60 seconds
Score 1: At least one episode of breathing lasting for 30-60 seconds
Score 0: No episodes of fetal breathing lasting for at least 30 seconds

Fetal tone

Ultrasound examination is carried out for a maximum of 30 minutes and a score is given according to the presence of movements in the extremities and spine.

Score 2: At least one episode of extension followed by flexion of extremities AND spine
Score 1: At least one episode of extension followed by flexion of extremities OR spine
Score 0: No episode of extension followed by flexion of extremities OR spine. The extremities are extended and the hands are open

Amniotic fluid volume

The amniotic fluid volume is assessed by ultrasound examination and measurement of a vertical pool.

Score 2: A pocket of fluid at least 2 cm deep
Score 1: A pocket of fluid 1-2 cm deep
Score 0: No pocket of fluid at least 1 cm deep

Placental grading

The placental appearance is evaluated by ultrasound examination.

Score 2: Smooth chorionic plate
Score 1: Placenta posterior and unable to evaluate
Score 0: Indentations of chorionic plate with echogenic areas

---

Table 3.14. Incidences of abnormal fetal biophysical profile score (BPS), fetal tachycardia, reduced fetal heart rate variation, non-reactive non-stress test and reduced amniotic fluid index (AFI) in patients with preterm prelabour amniorrhexis and positive or negative amniotic fluid or fetal blood cultures (Carroll *et al* 1995e).

Parameter	Amniotic fluid		Fetal blood	
	+ ve	- ve	+ ve	- ve
BPS score (<7/12)	36%	22%	50%	26%
Fetal heart rate (>95th centile)	14%	4%	28%	3%
Fetal heart rate variability (<5th centile)	28%	15%	36%	15%
Non-reactive non-stress test	39%	63%	50%	59%
AFI (< 5 cm)	82%	78%	100%	23%

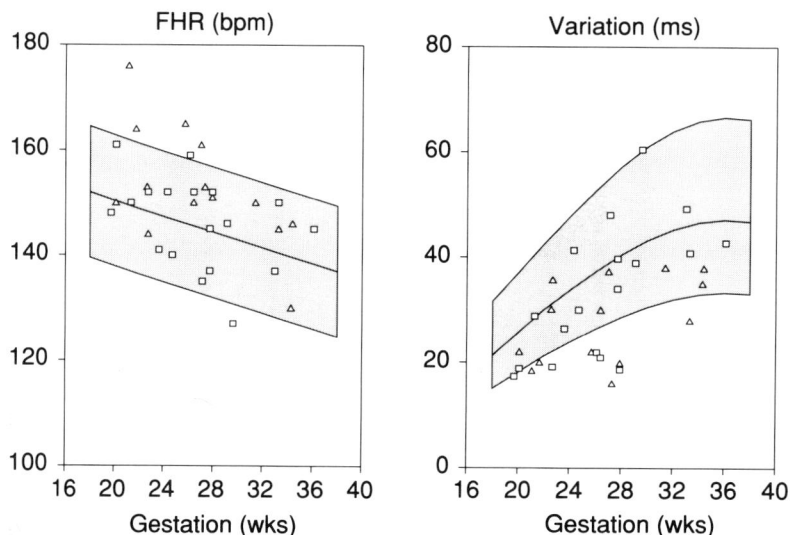

Figure 3.7. Baseline fetal heart rate (FHR) and fetal heart rate variation in pregnancies with preterm prelabour amniorrhexis and positive fetal blood cultures (Δ) or positive amniotic fluid cultures (□), plotted on the appropriate reference range with gestation (mean, 5th and 95th centiles). Adapted from Carroll *et al* (1995e).

Amniotic fluid volume

In normal pregnancy the volume of amniotic fluid increases from approximately 250 mL at 20 weeks of gestation to a maximum of around 1000 mL at 36 weeks; thereafter the volume gradually decreases (Queenan *et al* 1972).

Biophysical profile score

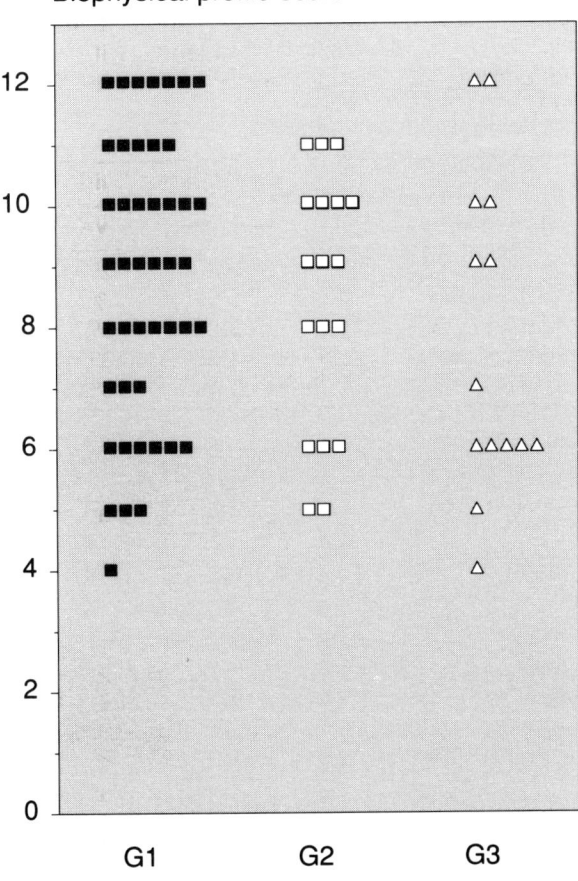

Figure 3.8. Biophysical profile score (BPS) in pregnancies with preterm prelabour amniorrhexis. The diagnosis of intrauterine infection was made on the basis of positive amniotic fluid and/or fetal blood cultures. In group 1 (G1) amniotic fluid and fetal blood cultures were negative, in group 2 (G2) amniotic fluid cultures were positive and in group 3 (G3) fetal blood cultures were positive. Adapted from Carroll *et al* (1995e).

In preterm prelabour amniorrhexis, the amniotic fluid volume is inevitably decreased and the decrease is more marked in those with intrauterine infection. This has been shown in a study measuring the amniotic fluid index (Table 3.15, Figure 3.9; Carroll *et al* 1995e) and in two others that measured the vertical diameter of the largest pocket of amniotic fluid (Vintzileos *et al* 1985a, 1986b). However, assessment of amniotic fluid volume does not provide sensitive prediction of intrauterine infection (Table 3.16)

Table 3.15. Measurement of amniotic fluid index according to Moore *et al* (1990).

Amniotic fluid index
• Patient placed in the supine position
• Uterus viewed as four equal quadrants
• Ultrasound transducer perpendicular to plane of the floor and aligned longitudinally with the patient's spine
• Vertical depth of the largest clear amniotic fluid pocket is measured in mm
• Amniotic fluid index = sum of four quadrant pocket depths

Table 3.16. True positive rate (TP) and false positive rate (FP) of low amniotic fluid volume, in the prediction of intrauterine infection in patients with preterm prelabour amniorrhexis. The criteria for the diagnosis of infection included clinical signs and/or neonatal sepsis (*), or positive amniotic fluid culture (+ve AFC). VD = vertical diameter of largest pool of amniotic fluid; AFI = amniotic fluid index

Author	Test	N	Criteria	TP	FP
Vintzileos *et al* 1986b	VD <1 cm	54	Clinical*	50%	7%
Miller *et al* 1990	VD <1 cm	47	Clinical	0%	34%
Gauthier *et al* 1992	VD <2 cm	111	+ve AFC	43%	19%
Goldstein *et al* 1989	VD <1 cm	41	+ve AFC	77%	34%
Carroll *et al* 1995e	AFI <5 cm	89	+ve AFC	82%	78%
Carroll *et al* 1995e	AFI <1 cm	41	+ve FBC	100%	23%

One possible explanation for the finding that, in the presence of infection, the amniotic fluid volume is less than in those without infection, is that amniotic fluid contains antimicrobial factors and consequently a decrease in fluid volume reduces the inherent ability to prevent intrauterine infection. However, this hypothesis implies that infection is secondary to amniorrhexis and recent evidence suggests that infection may be the cause rather than the consequence of amniorrhexis (see Chapter 2).

An alternative explanation for the association between low amniotic fluid volume and infection is that the extent of membrane rupture and therefore the amount of fluid loss is greater when the underlying mechanism of amniorrhexis is infection.

Doppler studies of the placental and fetal circulation

Doppler studies of the umbilical arterial circulation in pregnancies with chorioamnionitis have provided conflicting results with some

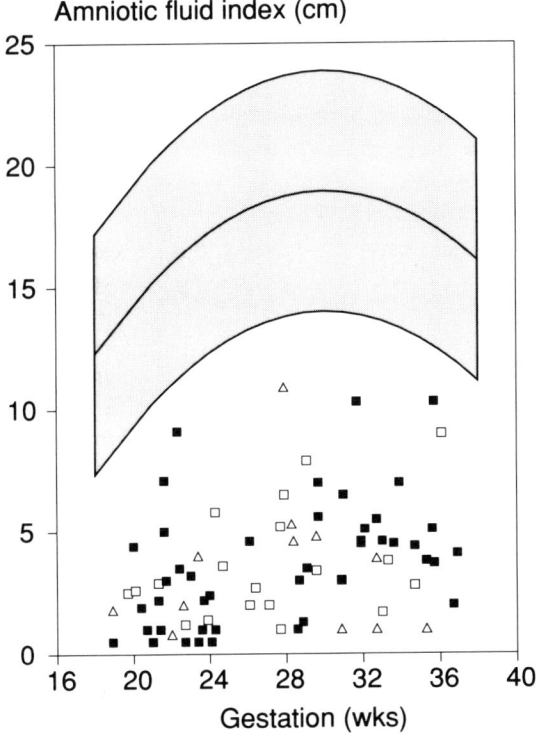

Figure 3.9. Amniotic fluid index in pregnancies with preterm prelabour amniorrhexis plotted on the appropriate reference range with gestation (mean, 5th and 95th centiles). The diagnosis of intrauterine infection was made on the basis of positive amniotic fluid and/or fetal blood cultures. In group 1 (■) amniotic fluid and fetal blood cultures were negative, in group 2 (□) amniotic fluid cultures were positive and in group 3 (Δ) fetal blood cultures were positive. Adapted from Carroll *et al* (1995e).

reporting an increase and others no change in impedence to flow (Brar *et al* 1989, Fleming *et al* 1991, Abramowicz *et al* 1992, Leo *et al* 1992).

In two cross sectional studies, involving a total of 35 patients with clinical chorioamnionitis, impedance to flow in the umbilical arteries was always normal (Brar *et al* 1989, Leo *et al* 1992).

In a longitudinal study of 22 patients with preterm prelabour amniorrhexis and umbilical vasculitis, although there was an increase of impedance in the umbilical arteries 24 hours before delivery compared to previous measurements, impedance had remained within the normal range (Fleming *et al* 1991). In another longitudinal study of uterine and umbilical arteries in 60 patients with amniorrhexis, including 12 who developed clinical chorioamnionitis, there was no significant increase in impedance even in measurements taken within 24 hours before delivery (Abramowicz *et al* 1992).

Carroll *et al* (1995f) performed Doppler studies immediately before cordocentesis and amniocentesis for bacteriological studies in 69 pregnancies with preterm prelabour amniorrhexis. The mean pulsatility indices in the uterine and umbilical arteries and in the fetal middle cerebral arteries and thoracic aorta were not significantly different from the appropriate normal mean for gestation and there were no significant differences between those with and without intrauterine infection (Figures 3.10 and 3.11).

These findings suggest that chorioamnionitis is not associated with a major degree of vasoconstriction in the uteroplacental or fetoplacental circulation. Consequently, Doppler does not provide

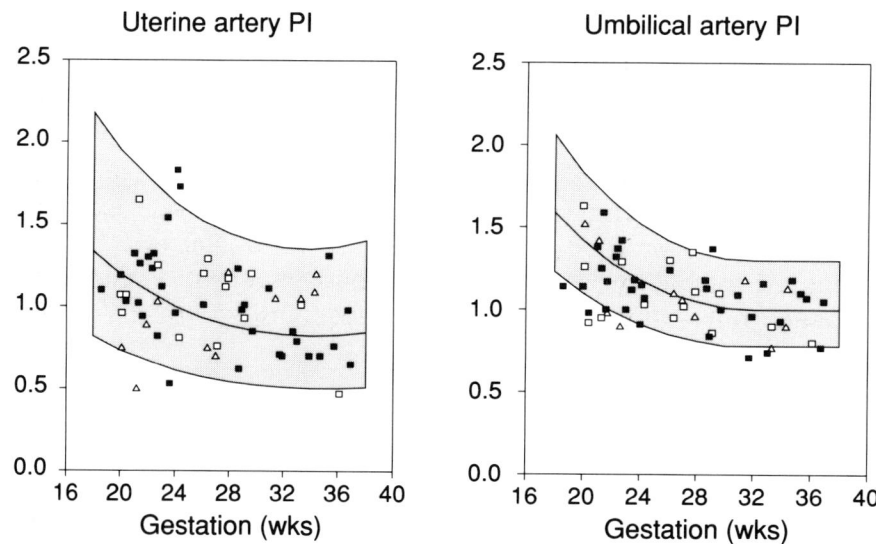

Figure 3.10. Pulsatility index (PI) of the uterine and umbilical arteries in pregnancies with preterm prelabour amniorrhexis plotted on the appropriate reference range with gestation (mean, 5th and 95th centiles). (■) negative amniotic fluid and fetal blood cultures, (□) positive amniotic fluid cultures, (Δ) positive fetal blood cultures. Adapted from Carroll *et al* (1995f).

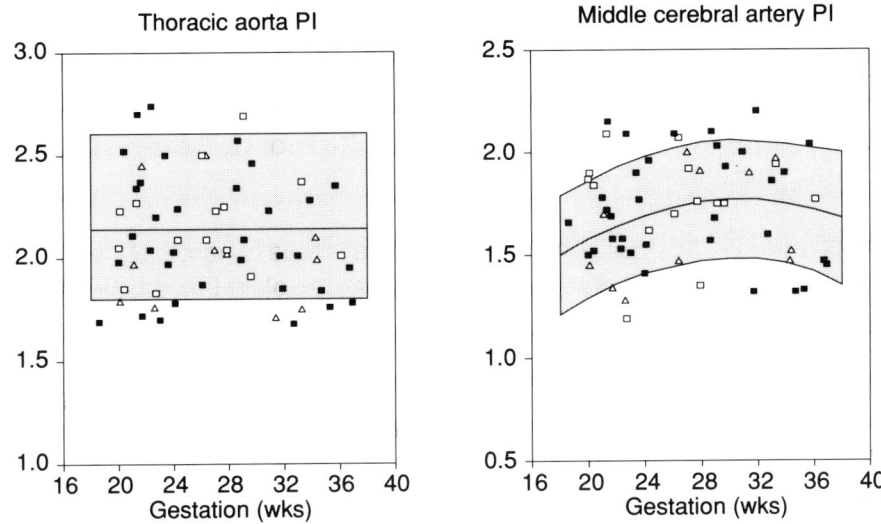

Figure 3.11. Pulsatility index (PI) of the fetal descending thoracic aorta and middle cerebral artery in pregnancies with preterm prelabour amniorrhexis plotted on the appropriate reference range with gestation (mean, 5th and 95th centiles). (■) negative amniotic fluid and fetal blood cultures, (□) positive amniotic fluid cultures, (△) positive fetal blood cultures. Adapted from Carroll *et al* (1995f).

a clinically useful distinction between infected and non-infected cases. However, Doppler studies in pregnancies with suspected amniorrhexis may be useful in the differential diagnosis from oligohydramnios due to uteroplacental insufficiency and intrauterine growth retardation. In the latter there is an increase in impedance to flow in the uterine and/or umbilical arteries with decreased pulsatility index in the fetal cerebral vessels and increased pulsatility index in the descending thoracic aorta (Bilardo *et al* 1990).

Fetal blood gases

Cordocentesis in pregnancies with preterm prelabour amniorrhexis has demonstrated that the mean umbilical venous blood pO_2 and pH are not significantly different from the appropriate normal mean for gestation and there are no significant differences between those with positive or negative fetal blood and amniotic fluid cultures (Figure 3.12). These findings demonstrate that, in the presence of intrauterine infection, fetal oxygenation is not impaired and are consistent with those of previous studies that examined umbilical cord blood obtained after delivery in patients with clinical chorioamnionitis or positive neonatal blood cultures (Vintzileos *et al* 1985b, Hankins *et al* 1991, Meyer *et al* 1992).

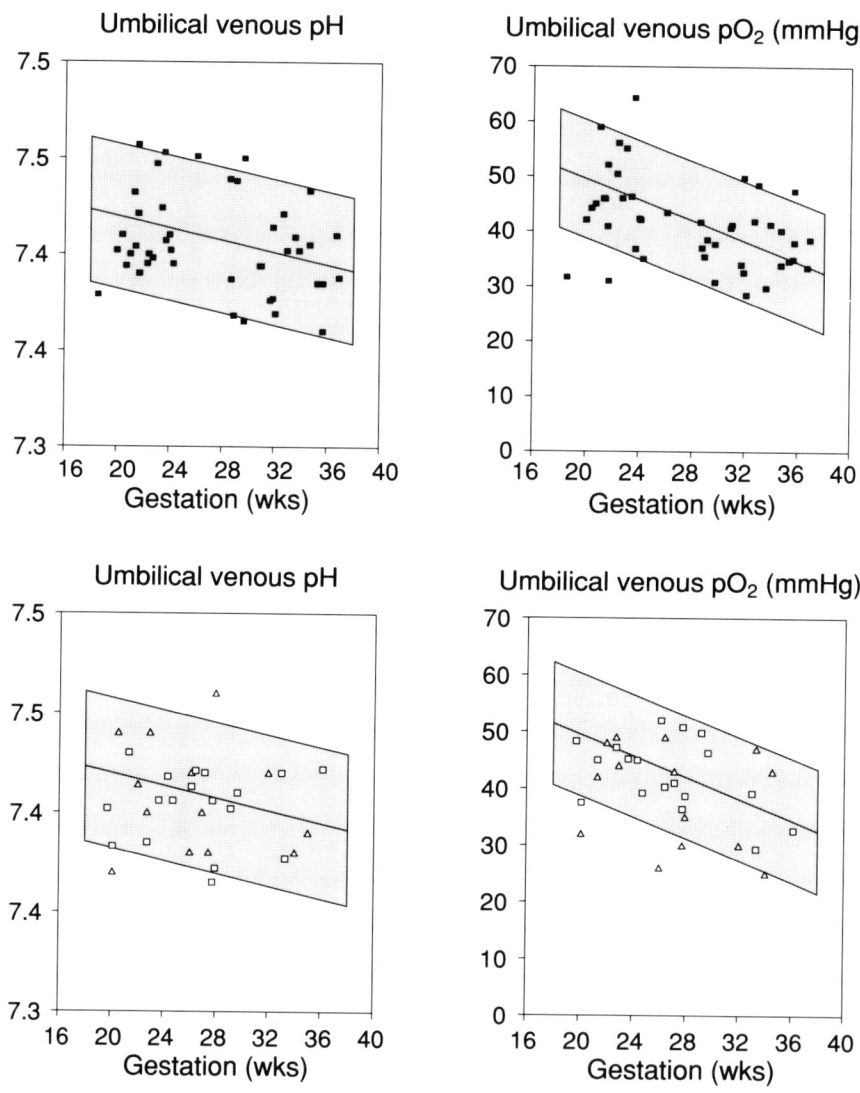

Figure 3.12. Umbilical venous blood pH and pO_2 in pregnancies with preterm prelabour amniorrhexis plotted on the appropriate reference range with gestation (mean, 5th and 95th centiles). On the top are those with negative amniotic fluid and fetal blood cultures, on the bottom are those with positive amniotic fluid (□) or fetal blood (Δ) cultures. Adapted from Carroll *et al* 1995e.

CONCLUSIONS

The diagnosis of intrauterine infection is made by culture of amniotic fluid and fetal blood. However, the results of culture may not be ready in time for purposeful obstetric intervention because pregnancies with infection deliver within a few days of amniorrhexis. This problem is partly overcome with the use of rapid tests to predict the presence of infection, the most useful of which are amniotic fluid Gram stain and fetal blood leukocyte count.

In the majority of pregnancies with preterm prelabour amniorrhexis and positive amniotic fluid or fetal blood cultures, the infection is subclinical. Consequently, the observations of normal maternal temperature, heart rate, leukocyte count and C-reactive protein should not reassure the attending physicians that there is no intrauterine infection. Similarly, the results of cultures of swabs from the lower genital tract do not provide sensitive prediction of intrauterine infection and they have a high false positive rate.

In pregnancies with amniorrhexis and intrauterine infection, placental perfusion and fetal oxygenation are normal. Consequently, currently available non-invasive methods for assessment of the fetus will not help distinguish between those with and without infection because these tests are designed to detect fetal responses to hypoxia.

REFERENCES

Abramowicz JS, Sherer DM, Warsof SL, Levy DL. Fetoplacental and uteroplacental Doppler blood flow velocity analysis in premature rupture of membranes. Am J Perinatol 1992;9:353-6.

Alger LS, Lovchik JC, Hebel JR, Blackmon LR, Crenshaw MC. The association of Chlamydia trachomatis, Neisseria gonorrhoea, and Group B streptococci with preterm rupture of the membranes and pregnancy outcome. Am J Obstet Gynecol 1988;159:397-404.

Altura BM, Malaviya AD, Reich CF, Orkin LR. Effects of vasoactive agents on isolated human umbilical arteries and veins. Am J Physiol 1972;222:345-55.

Berman SM, Harrison RH, Boyce WT, Haffner WJ, Lewis M, Arthur JB. Low birth weight, prematurity, and postpartum endometritis. JAMA 1987;257:1189-94.

Bilardo CM, Nicolaides KH, Campbell S. Doppler measurements of fetal and uteroplacental circulation: relationship with umbilical venous blood gases measured at cordocentesis. Am J Obstet Gynecol 1990;162:115-20.

Bjoro K, Stray-Pedersen S. Effects of vasoactive autacoids on different segments of human umbilicoplacental vessels. Gynecol Obstet Invest1986;22: 1-6.

Bobitt JR, Damato JD, Sakakini J. Perinatal complications in Group B streptococcal carriers: A longitudinal study of prenatal patients. Am J Obstet Gynecol 1985;151:711-17.

Brar HS, Medearis AL, Platt LD. Relationship of systolic/diastolic ratios from umbilical velocimetry to fetal heart rate. Am J Obstet Gynecol 1989;160:188-91.

Broekhuizen FF, Gilman M, Hamilton PR. Amniocentesis for gram stain and culture in preterm premature rupture of the membranes. Obstet Gynecol 1985;66:316-21.

Carey JC, Blackwelder WC, Nugent RP, Matteson MA, Rao AV, Eschenbach DA, Lee MLF, Rettig PJ, Regan JA, Geromanos KL, Martin DH, Pastorek JG, Gibbs RS, Lipscomb KA. Antepartum cultures for Ureaplasma urealyticum are not useful in predicting pregnancy outcome. Am J Obstet Gynecol 1991;164:728-33.

Carroll SG, Philpott-Howard J, Nicolaides KH. Amniotic fluid Gram stain and leucocyte count in the prediction of intrauterine infection in preterm prelabour amniorhexis. Fetal Diag Ther 1995a (In press).

Carroll SG, Nicolaides KH. Fetal hematological response to intrauterine infection in preterm prelabour amniorrhexis. Fetal Diag Ther 1995b (In press).

Carroll SG, Papaioannou S, Davies ET, Nicolaides KH. Maternal assessment in the prediction of intrauterine infection in preterm prelabour amniorrhexis. Fetal Diag Ther 1995c (In press).

Carroll SG, Papaioannou S, Ntumazah IL, Philpott-Howard J, Nicolaides KH. Lower genital tract swabs in the prediction of intrauterine infection in preterm prelabour amniorrhexis. Br J Obstet Gynaecol 1995d (In press).

Carroll SG, Papaioannou S, Nicolaides KH. Assessment of fetal activity and amniotic fluid volume in pregnancies complicated by preterm prelabour amniorrhexis. Am J Obstet Gynecol 1995e;172:1427-35.

Carroll SG, Papaioannou S, Nicolaides KH. Doppler studies of the placental and fetal circulation in pregnancies with preterm prelabour amniorrhexis. Ultrasound Obstet Gynecol 1995f;5:184-8.

Cassell G.H., Waites K.B., Watson H.L., Crouse D.T., Harawawa R. Ureaplasma urealyticum intrauterine infection: Role in prematurity and disease in newborns. Clin Microbiol Rev 1993;6:69-87.

Cassell GH, Waiters KB, Gibbs RS, Davis JK. Role of Ureaplasma urealyticum in amnionitis. Pediatr Infect Dis J 1986;5:247-52.

Christensen RD, Macfarlane JL, Taylor NL, Hill HR, Rothstein G. Blood and marrow neutrophils during experimental Group B streptococcal infection: Quantification of the stem cell, proliferative, storage and circulating pools. Pediatr Res 1982;16:549-53.

Christensen RD, Rothstein G. Exhaustion of mature marrow neutrophils in neonates with sepsis. J Pediatr 1980a;96:316-18.

Christensen RD, Rothstein G. Efficiency of neutrophil migration in the neonate. Pediatr Res 1980b;14:1147-9.

Cotton DB, Hill LM, Strassner HT, Platt LD, Ledger WJ. Use of amniocentesis in preterm gestation with ruptured membranes. Obstet Gynecol 1984;63:38-48.

Coultrip L.L., Grossman J.H. Evaluation of rapid diagnostic tests in the detection of microbial invasion of the amniotic cavity. Am J Obstet Gynecol 1992;167:1231-42.

Dadd A.H., Dagnall V.P., Everall P.H., Jones A.C. The survival of Streptococcus pyogenes on bacteriological swabs made from various fibres. J Med Microbiol 1970; 3:561-72.

Davies NP, Buggins AGS, Snijders RJM, Jenkins E, Layton DM, Nicolaides KH. Blood leucocyte count in the human fetus. Arch Dis Child 1992;67:399-402.

Del Valle GO, Joffe GM, Izquierdo LA, Smith JF, Gilson GJ, Curet LB. The biophysical profile and the nonstress test: Poor predictors of chorioamnionitis and fetal infection in prolonged preterm premature rupture of membranes. Obstet Gynecol 1992;80:106-10.

Elin RJ, Hosseini J. Clinical utility of the *Limulus* amebocyte lysate test. Bacterial endotoxin, structure, biomedical significance and detection with the *Limulus* amebocyte lysate test. In: ten Cate JW, Buller HR, Sturk A, Levin J, eds. Progress in clinical and biological research. New York: Alan R Liss, 1985:307-24.

Ernest JM, Swain M, Block SM, Nelson LH, Hatjis CG, Meis PJ. C-reactive protein: A limited test for managing patients with preterm labour or preterm rupture of membranes? Am J Obstet Gynecol 1987;156:449-54.

Evans M, Hajj SN, Devoe LD, Angerman NS, Moawad AH. C-reactive protein as a predictor of infectious morbidity with premature rupture of membranes. Am J Obstet Gynecol 1980;138:648-52.

Farb HF, Arnesen M, Geistler P, Knox E. C-reactive protein with premature rupture of membranes and premature labour. Obstet Gynecol 1983;62:49-51.

Ferguson MG, Rhodes PG, Morrison JC, Puckett CM. Clinical amniotic fluid infection and its effect on the neonate. Am J Obstet Gynecol 1985;151:1058-61.

Fisk NM. A dipstick test for infection in preterm premature rupture of the membranes. J Perin Med 1987;15:565-8.

Fleming AD, Salafia CM, Vintzileos AM, Rodis JF, Campbell WA, Bantham F. The relationships among umbilical artery velocimetry, fetal biophysical profile, and placental inflammation in preterm premature rupture of the membranes. Am J Obstet Gynecol 1991;164:38-41.

Garite TJ, Freeman RK, Linzey M, Braly P. The use of amniocentesis in patients with premature rupture of membranes. Obstet Gynecol 1979;54:226-30.

Garite TJ, Freeman RK. Chorioamnionitis in the preterm gestation. Obstet Gynecol 1982;59:539-45.

Gauthier DW, Meyer WJ, Bieniarz A. Biophysical profile as a predictor of amniotic fluid culture results. Obstet Gynecol 1992;80:102-5.

Gauthier DW, Meyer WJ, Bieniarz A. Correlation of amniotic fluid glucose concentration and intraamniotic infection in patients with preterm labour or premature rupture of membranes. Am J Obstet Gynecol 1991;165:1150-61.

Gerdes JS. Clinicopathologic approach to the diagnosis of neonatal sepsis. Clin Perinat 1991;18:361-81.

Gewolb IH, Hobbins JC, Tan SY. Amniotic fluid cortisol in high-risk human pregnancies. Obstet Gynecol 1977;49:466-70.

Goldstein I, Copel JA, Hobbins JC. Fetal behaviour in preterm premature rupture of the membranes. Clin Perinat 1989;16:735-55.

Gravett MG, Eschenbach DA, Speigel-Brown CA, Holmes KK. Rapid diagnosis of amniotic fluid infection by gas-liquid chromatography. N Eng J Med 1982;306:725-8.

Guzick DS, Winn K. The association of chorioamnionitis with preterm delivery. Obstet Gynecol. 1985;65:11-15.

Hankins GDV, Snyder RR, Yeomans ER. Umbilical arterial and venous acid-base and blood gas values and the effect of chorioamnionitis on those values in a cohort of preterm infants. Am J Obstet Gynecol 1991;164:1261-4.

Hardy PH, Nell EE, Spence MR, Hardy JB, Graham DA, Rosenbaum RC. Prevalence of six sexually transmitted disease agents among pregnant inner-city adolescents and pregnancy outcome. Lancet 1984;2:333-7.

Harrison RF, Hurley R, deLouvois J. Genital mycoplasmas and birth weight in offspring of primigravid women. Am J Obstet Gynecol 1979;133:201-3.

Harrison RH, Alexander ER, Weinstein L, Lewis M, Nash M, Sim D. Cervical Chlamydia trachomatis and mycoplasmal infections in pregnancy. JAMA 1983;250: 1721-7.

Hawrylyshyn P, Bernstein P, Milligan JE, Soldin S, Pollard A, Papsin FR. Premature rupture of membranes: The role of C-reactive protein in the prediction of chorioamnionitis. Am J Obstet Gynecol 1983;147:240-6.

Hellerqvist CG, Rojas J, Green RS, Sell S, Sundell H, Stahlman MT. Studies of group B, beta-hemolytic streptococcus. Isolation and partial characterization of an extracellular toxin. Pediatr Res 1981;15:892-8.

Hess LW, O'Brien WF, Holmberg JA, Winkler CA, Monaghan WP, Hemming VG. Plasma and amniotic fluid concentrations of fibronectin during normal pregnancy. Obstet Gynecol 1986;68:25-8.

Hill HR, Shigeoka AO, Augustine NH, Pritchard D, Lundbho JL, Schwarz RS. Fibronectin enhances the opsonic and protective activity of momoclonal and polyclonal antibody against group B streptococci. J Exp Med 1984;159:1618-28.

Hillier SL, Krohn MA, Nugent RP, Gibbs RS. Characteristics of three vaginal flora patterns assessed by Gram stain among pregnant women. Am J Obstet Gynecol 1992;166:938-44.

Hillier SL, Martius J, Krohn M, Kiviat N, Holmes KK, Eschenbach DA. A case control study of chorioamniotic infection and histologic chorioamnionitis in prematurity. NEJM 1988;319:972-8.

Hillier SL, Witkin SS, Krohn MA, Watts DH, Kiviat NB, Eschenbach DA. The relationship of amniotic fluid cytokines and preterm delivery, amniotic fluid infection, histologic chorioamnionitis, and chorioamnion infection. Obstet Gynecol 1993;81:941-8.

Howard RB, Hosokawa T, Maguire MH. Pressor and depressor actions of prostanoids in the intact human feto-placental vascular bed. Prostaglandins Leukotrienes Med 1986;21:323-30.

Hyde S, Smotherman J, Moore J, Altshulter G. A model of bacterially induced umbilical vein spasm, relevant to fetal hypoperfusion. Obstet Gynecol 1989;73:966-70.

Ismail A, Zinaman MJ, Lowensohn RI, Moawad AH. The significance of C-reactive protein levels in women with premature rupture of membranes. Am J Obstet Gynecol 1985;151:541-4.

Katz VL, Moos MK, Cefalo RC, Thorp JM, Bowes W.A., Wells S.D. Group B streptococci: Results of a protocol of antepartum screening and intrapartum treatment. Am J Obstet Gynecol 1994;170:521-6.

Klein JO. Mycoplasma infections. In Remington JS, Klein LO, eds. Infectious diseases of the fetus and newborn infant. 3rd ed. Philadelphia: WB Saunders, 1990:446-63.

Kornman L, Jacobs V, Hodgson RP, Godfrey J, Dunlevy L, Tyler JPP, Baird PJ, Hudson CN.. Chorioamnionitis: How useful is the determination of C-reactive protein? Aust NZ J Obstet Gynaecol 1988;28:45-8.

Kusimi RK, Grover PJ, Kunin CM. Rapid detection of pyuria by leukocyte estrase activity. JAMA 1981;245:1653-4.

Lamont RF, Taylor-Robinson D, Newman M, Wigglesworth J, Elder MG. Spontaneous early preterm labour associated with abnormal genital bacterial colonization. Br J Obstet Gynaecol 1986;93:804-10.

Leo MV, Skurnick JH, Ganesh VV, Adhate A, Apuzzio JJ. Clinical chorioamnionitis is not predicted by umbilical artery doppler velocimetry in patients with premature of membranes. Obstet Gynecol 1992;79:916-18.

Mak KK, Gude NM, Walters WAW, Boura ALA. Effects of vasoactive autacoids on the human umbilical-fetal placental vasculature. Br J Obstet Gynaecol 1984;91: 99-106.

McDonald H, Vigneswaran R, O'Loughlin JA Group B streptococcal colonization and preterm labour. Aust NZ J Obstet Gynaecol 1989;29:291-93.

McDonald HM, O'Loughlin JA, Jolley P, Vigneswaran R, McDonald PJ. Prenatal microbial risk factors associated with preterm birth. Br J Obstet Gynaecol 1992;99:190-6.

McGregor JA, French JI, Richter R, Vuchetich M, Bachus V, Seo K, Hillier S, Judson FN, McFee J, Schoonmaker J, Todd J. Cervicovaginal microflora and pregnancy outcome: Results of a double-blind, placebo-controlled trial of erythromycin treatment. Am J Obstet Gynecol 1990;163:1580-91.

Meyer BA, Dickinson JE, Chambers C, Parisi VM. The effect of fetal sepsis on umbilical cord blood gases. Am J Obstet Gynecol 1992;166:612-17.

Miller JM, Kho MS, Brown HL, Gabert HA. Clinical chorioamnionitis is not predicted by an ultrasonic biophysical profile in patients with premature rupture of membranes. Obstet Gynecol 1990;76:1051-3.

Minkoff H, Grunebaum AN, Schwarz RH, Feldman J, Cummings M, Crombleholme W, Clark L, Pringle G, McCormack WM. Risk factors for prematurity and premature rupture of membranes: A prospective study of the vaginal flora in pregnancy. Am J Obstet Gynecol 1984;150:965-72.

Moore TR, Cayle JE. The amniotic fluid index in normal human pregnancy. Am J Obstet Gynecol 1990;162:1168-73.

Mueller-Heubach E, Rubinstein DN, Schwarz SS. Histologic chorioamnionitis and preterm delivery in different patient populations. Obstet Gynecol 1990;75:622-6.

O'Brien WF, Knuppel RA, Morales WJ, Angel JL, Torres CT. Amniotic fluid alpha 1-antitrypsin concentration in premature rupture of the membranes. Am J Obstet Gynecol 1990;162:756-9.

Pankuch GA, Applebaum PC, Lorenz RP, Botti JJ, Schachter J, Naeye RL. Placental microbiology and histology and the pathogenesis of chorioamnionitis. Obstet Gynecol 1984;64:802-6.

Perkins RP, Zhou S, Butler C, Skipper BJ. Histologic chorioamnionitis in pregnancies of various gestational ages: Implications in preterm rupture of membranes. Obstet Gynecol 1987;70:856-60.

Potter NT, Kosuda L, Bigazzi PE, Fleming AD, Vintzileos AM, Homon C, Salafia CM. Relationships among cytokines (IL-1, TNF, and IL-8) and histologic markers of acute ascending intrauterine infection. J Matern Fetal Med 1992;1:142-7.

Queenan JT, Thompson W, Whitfield CR, Shah SI. Amniotic fluid volumes in normal pregnancies. Am J Obstet Gynecol 1972;114:34-8.

Quinn PA, Buatany J, Taylor J, Hannah W. Chrioamnionitis: Its association with pregnancy outcome and microbial infection. Am J Obstet Gynecol 1987;156:379-87.

Robert JA, Romero R, Costigan K. Amniotic fluid concentrations of fibronectin and intra-amniotic infection. Am J Perinatol 1988;5:26-8.

Romem Y, Artal R. C-reactive protein as a predictor for chorioamnionitis in cases of premature of the membranes. Am J Obstet Gynecol 1984;150:546-50.

Romero R, Brody DT, Oyarzun E, Mazor M, King Wu Y, Hobbins JC, Durum SK. Interleukin-1: A signal for the onset of parturition. Am J Obstet Gynecol 1989;160:1117-23.

Romero R, Emamian M, Wan M, Yarkoni S, McCormack W, Mazor M, Hobbins JC. The value of the leukocyte esterase test in diagnosing intra-amniotic infection. Am J Perinatol 1988a;5:64-9.

Romero R, Scharf K, Mazor M, Emamian M, Hobbins JC. The clinical value of gas-liquid chromatography in the detection of intra-amniotic microbial invasion. Obstet Gynecol 1988b;72;44-50.

Romero R, Quintero R, Oyarzun E, King Wu Y, Sabo V, Mazor M, Hobbins JC. Intraamniotic infection and the onset of labour in preterm premature rupture of the membranes. Am J Obstet Gynecol 1988c;159:661-6.

Romero R, Kadar N, Hobbins JC, Duff GW. Infection and labour: The detection of endotoxin in amniotic fluid. Am J Obstet Gynecol 1987;157:815-19.

Romero R, Mazor M, Sepulveda W, Avila C, Copeland D, Williams J. Tumor necrosis factor in preterm and term labour. Am J Obstet Gynecol 1992;166:1576-87.

Romero R, Salafia CM, Athanassiadis AP, Hanaoka S, Mazor M, Sepulveda W, Bracken MB. The relationship between acute infammatory lesions of the preterm placenta and amniotic fluid microbiology. Am J Obstet Gynecol 1992;166:1382-8.

Romero R, Yoon BH, Mazor M, Gomez R, Gonzalez R, Diamond MP, Baumann P, Araneda H, Kenney JS, Cotton DB, Sehgal P. A comparitive study of the diagnostic performance of amniotic fluid glucose, white blood cell count, interleukin-6, and Gram stain in the detection of microbial invasion in patients with premature rupture of membranes. Am J Obstet Gynecol 1993;169:839-51.

Roussis P, Rosemond RL, Glass C, Boehm F. Preterm premature rupture of membranes: Detection of infection. Am J Obstet Gynecol 1991;165:1099-104.

Sandberg K, Englehardt B, Hellerqvist C, Sundell H. Pulmonary response to group B streptococcal toxin in young lambs. J Appl Physiol 1987;63:2024-30.

Schlievert P., Larsen B., Johnson W. Bacterial growth inhibition by amniotic fluid. Demonstration of the variability of bacterial growth inhibition by amniotic fluid with a new platelet-count technique. Am J Obstet Gynecol 1975;122:809-13.

Seo K, McGregor JA, French JI. Preterm birth is associated with increased risk of maternal and neonatal infection. Obstet Gynecol 1992;79:75-80.

Svensson L, Ingemarsson I, Mardh P. Chorioamnionitis and the isolation of organisms from the placenta. Obstet Gynecol. 1986;67:403-9.

Sweet RL, Landers DV, Walker C, Schachter J. Chlamydia trachomatis infection and pregnancy outcome. Am J Obstet Gynecol 1987;156:824-33.

Van De Water III L: Phagocytosis. In Jan McDonagh (ed): Haematology, vol 5; Plasma Fibronectin: Structure and Function. New York: Marcel Dekker 1985:175-98.

Vintzileos AM, Campbell WA, Ingardia CJ, Nochimson DJ. The fetal biophysical profile and its predictive value. Obstet Gynecol 1983;62:271-8.

Vintzileos AM, Winston WA, Nochimson DJ, Weinbaum PJ. Degree of oligohydramnios and pregnancy outcome in patients with premature rupture of the membranes. Obstet Gynecol 1985a;66:162-7.

Vintzileos AM, Campbell WA, Nochimson DJ, Connolly ME, Fuenfer MM, Hoehn GJ. The fetal biophysical profile in patients with premature rupture of the membranes- An early prediction of fetal infection. Am J Obstet Gynecol 1985b;152:510-16.

Vintzileos AM, Campbell WA, Nochimson DJ, Weinbaum PJ, Mirochnick MH, Escoto DT. Fetal biophysical profile versus amniocentesis in predicting infection in preterm premature rupture of the membranes. Obstet Gynecol 1986a;68:488-94.

Vintzileos AM, Campbell WA, Nochimson DJ, Weinbaum PJ, Escoto DT, Mirochnick MH. Qualitative amniotic fluid volume versus amniocentesis in predicting infection in preterm premature rupture of the membranes. Obstet Gynecol 1986b;67:579-83.

Vonsee HJ, Stobberingh EE, Bouckaert PXJM, de Haan J, van Boven CPA. Detection of Chlamydia trachomatis, *Mycoplasma hominis* and *Ureaplasma urealyticum* in pregnant Dutch women. Eur J Obstet Gynecol 1989;32:149-56.

Watts DH, Krohn MA, Hillier SL, Wener MH, Kiviat NB, Eschenbach DA. Characteristics of women in preterm labour asssociated with elevated C-reactive protein levels. Obstet Gynecol 1993;82:509-14.

Weiss PAM, Hoffman H, Winter R, Parstner P, Lichtenegger W. Amniotic fluid glucose values in normal and abnormal pregnancies. Obstet Gynecol 1985;65: 333-9.

Wientzen R.L. Genital Mycoplasmas and the pediatrician. Pediatr Infect Dis J 1990;9:232-5.

Zlatnick FJ, Gellhaus TM, Banda JA, Koontz FP, Burmeister LF. Histologic chorioamnionitis, microbial infection and prematurity. Obstet Gynecol. 1990;76:355-9.

Preterm prelabour amniorrhexis: management considerations

DIAGNOSIS AND TREATMENT OF AMNIORRHEXIS

Amniotic fluid in the vagina

The presence of a pool of fluid in the vagina at speculum examination is highly suggestive of amniorrhexis, but a series of tests have been used to confirm that this is indeed amniotic fluid (Table 4.1).

Gold (1927) used a litmus paper to detect the change in pH of vaginal fluid from normal acidic to alkaline, due to the presence of amniotic fluid. The Nitrazine test, which also detects pH change, but more accurately than litmus paper over the physiological range, was introduced in the 1930s and is still the most widely used test today (Baptisti 1938, Abe 1940). Other tests utilised microscopic examination of the vaginal fluid to demonstrate the presence of (i) lanugo hair (Volet *et al* 1960), (ii) fetal fat particles, stained with sudan III (Von Numers 1936), (iii) fetal epithelial cells, stained with Nile blue (Brosens & Gordon 1965), pinocyanole chloride (Averette *et al* 1963) or acridine orange (Kushner *et al* 1964), and (iv) a characteristic ferning of the crystallisation pattern of dried amniotic fluid due to its sodium chloride and protein content (Paalova 1958, Volet 1960).

Table 4.1. Tests used for the detection of amniotic fluid in the vagina reporting the true positive (TP) and false positive (FP) rates.

Author	Test	TP	FP
Berlind 1932, King 1935	Bromthymol blue	96%	1%
Von Numers 1936	Fetal fat	96%	3%
Baptisti 1938, Abe 1940	Nitrazine	95%	2%
Paavola 1958	Ferning	96%	3%
Volet *et al* 1960	Lanugo hair	2%	-
Averette *et al* 1963	Pinacynol	97%	3%
Kushner *et al* 1964	Acridine orange	90%	14%
Brosens & Gordon 1965	Nile blue	98%	0%
Rochelson *et al* 1987	Alphafetoprotein	98%	?
Eriksen *et al* 1992	Fetal fibronectin	98%	73%
Lockwood *et al* 1994	ILGF-1	75%	7%

A study evaluating the various tests in the diagnosis of amniorrhexis examined 100 consecutive women in labour with either intact or ruptured membrane (Friedman & McElin 1969). The best results were obtained with the nitrazine and ferning tests; the sensitivity was around 90%, but this decreased as the time from amniorrhexis increased. The false positive rate was 17% for the nitrazine test, due to contamination with urine, blood, or semen, and 6% for the ferning test, due to contamination with cervical mucus. A similar sensitivity and false positive rate was achieved by obtaining a history of a gush of fluid from the vagina'.

Other tests developed more recently include the use of monoclonal antibody assays to measure alphafetoprotein (Rochelson *et al* 1987), fetal fibronectin (Eriksen *et al* 1992), or detection of Insulin like growth factor binding protein-1 (Lockwood *et al* 1994). Maternal oral phenazopyridine and colorimetric analysis of vaginal fluid has also been used (Meyer *et al* 1991). It is uncertain whether any of these tests will prove sufficiently useful to replace the Nitrazine test.

Ultrasound examination

In patients with amniorrhexis, ultrasound examination is essential for exclusion of major anomalies, estimation of fetal weight, determination of presentation, and placental localisation.

Differential diagnosis of oligohydramnios

In patients with suspected amniorrhexis, ultrasound examination may confirm the presence of oligohydramnios. The differential diagnosis would be (i) amniorrhexis, (ii) severe uteroplacental insufficiency with fetal growth retardation and invariably abnormal Doppler results in the umbilical or uterine arteries and fetal vessels, and (iii) obstructive uropathy, renal dysplasia or renal agenesis.

Distinction between renal agenesis and amniorrhexis may be difficult, because the adrenals may be mistaken for kidneys and vice-versa and in both conditions fetal biometry and placental or fetal Doppler results are usually normal. In such cases, further questioning of the patient may reveal a history of intermittent loss of fluid thought to be urine, episodes of vaginal bleeding, or recent increase in vaginal discharge. Additionally, prolonged ultrasound examination may demonstrate fetal bladder filling. Very rarely, when there is still uncertainty of the diagnosis, amnioinfusion may be considered; in cases of amniorrhexis, intra-amniotic injection of 100-200 mL of Hartmans solution will invariably cause vaginal loss of fluid within a few minutes. Injection of a water soluble dye, such as fluorescein, has also been advocated (Smith 1976), but this is not necessary.

Estimation of fetal weight

In pregnancies at risk of preterm delivery, estimation of fetal weight is important in decision making concerning management, since birth weight is of critical value in determining both survival and handicap (see Chapter 1).

The fetal weight can be calculated from formulas incorporating various combinations of measurements of fetal head, abdomen and limbs (Shepard *et al* 1982, Hadlock *et al* 1984).

In preterm prelabour amniorrhexis and consequent reduction in amniotic fluid volume, it is more difficult to get accurate measurements of the various fetal parts. Nevertheless, several ultrasonographic studies have reported that, in pregnancies with amniorrhexis, estimates of fetal weight are no less accurate than in pregnancies with normal amniotic fluid volume (Kho *et al* 1989, Valea *et al* 1990, Toohey *et al* 1991).

Vaginal examination

Speculum examination

In pregnancies with suspected preterm prelabour amniorrhexis, a sterile speculum examination will help confirm the diagnosis, assess cervical dilatation and enable the taking of cervico-vaginal swabs for bacteriological studies. In such patients, there is probably little benefit in performing a digital examination in addition to the speculum examination, but no controlled comparisons to establish the benefit or not of either method have been made (Chalmers *et al* 1992).

Two studies on cervical assessment of women in labour reported a good correlation between results obtained by digital vaginal examination and those with speculum examination by the same individuals (Munson *et al* 1985, Brown *et al* 1993).

Digital examination

In the presence of amniorrhexis, digital vaginal and cervical examination should probably be avoided. First, micro-organisms may be transported from the perineum and vagina into the cervix, thereby increasing the risk of intrauterine infection and its adverse sequelae of preterm delivery and neonatal sepsis. Secondly, cervical manipulation may cause release of prostaglandins and initiation of labour.

A retrospective study of women with preterm prelabour amniorrhexis reported that the latency period in those who had a vaginal examination was significantly shorter than if a sterile speculum examination only was performed (Lewis *et al* 1992).

Removal of cervical suture

Patients with a history of cervical incompetence leading to second trimester deliveries may have subsequent pregnancies treated by insertion of a cervical suture. Should preterm prelabour amniorrhexis occur with the cerclage in situ there is a theoretical risk that this foreign body may act as a nidus for infection. Yeast and Garite (1988) have demonstrated that, provided the suture is removed at presentation, the risk of infectious morbidity is not higher than in patients with amniorrhexis in the absence of a cervical suture.

Membrane rupture is also a common complication of inserting a cervical suture; amniorrhexis has been reported in up to 50% of cases following emergency cerclage and one third of these occur perioperatively (Wong *et al* 1993). The management of such patients is uncertain.

Need for hospitalisation and bed rest?

In the presence of intrauterine infection there is usually spontaneous delivery within five days of amniorrhexis (see Chapter 2). When there is no infection the pregnancy may be prolonged for several months. Traditionally, such patients are hospitalised for observation and they are often kept in bed with the aim of reducing the loss of amniotic fluid. Such management, despite its major cost both in economic terms for the health service and family disruption for the individual, is of unproven value. In addition it has the potential risks of causing thromboembolic complications and leading to infection with resistant organisms.

A recent study has demonstrated that many of the patients with preterm prelabour amniorrhexis who fulfil certain criteria (singleton pregnancy, cephalic presentation, more than 72 hours from amniorrhexis, no clinical evidence of infection, cervix less than 4 cm dilated) can be managed at home (Carlan *et al* 1993). Such management was not associated with increase in adverse maternal or neonatal outcomes compared to those that were hospitalised.

Bed rest is widely prescribed for pregnancies at high risk of a wide variety of complications. It is somehow felt that bed rest may improve 'placental perfusion' and help 'relax' the uterus. However, randomised studies have demonstrated that bed rest is not associated with a reduction in the incidence of preterm delivery, low birth weight or perinatal death in either women at risk of preterm delivery or those with other complications such as non-proteinuric hypertension (see Chapter 1).

Monitoring uterine activity

The pattern of uterine activity in pregnancies with preterm prelabour amniorrhexis is similar to that of women with intact membranes who later go on to develop preterm labour; within 24 hours of the onset of labour there is an increase in the frequency of contractions (Campbell *et al* 1991).

Although objective recording of uterine activity may detect increased contraction frequency earlier than maternal subjective assessment, the efficacy of this method of monitoring has not yet been established (see Chapter 1).

Resealing of amniotic membranes

Spontaneous

In approximately 2-3% of patients with preterm prelabour amniorrhexis there is apparent 'resealing' of the membranes; they stop leaking fluid from the vagina and amniotic fluid reaccumulates in the amniotic cavity. In this group the duration of pregnancy is longer and perinatal mortality is lower than in patients who continue to lose amniotic fluid.

Johnson *et al* (1990) identified 24 women with preterm prelabour amniorrhexis who subsequently stopped losing fluid from the vagina and the Nitrazine test became negative. The obstetric outcome in this group was compared to matched controls who also had confirmed preterm prelabour amniorrhexis, but continued to leak amniotic fluid vaginally until delivery. Although the mean gestation at the time of amniorrhexis was the same in the two groups (30 weeks), the mean gestation at delivery in the group that 'resealed' was 38 weeks compared to 31 weeks for the controls; the incidence of respiratory distress syndrome and length of hospital stay in the infants from the group that 'resealed' was also correspondingly lower.

Insertion of fibrin plaque

For patients who continue to lose amniotic fluid, one suggested option is to insert a cervical suture and then inject a 'fibrin glue' up the cervical canal. Application of the fibrin clot can interrupt the leakage of amniotic fluid, promoting regeneration of chorion and amnion and their close contact with the decidua; direct closure of the ruptured membranes is not attained.

In a study of 17 patients with preterm prelabour amniorrhexis at 18-32 weeks, prolongation of the pregnancy beyond 28 days from

1986). However, in this study there were no controls and it is uncertain whether this form of therapy is of any benefit to the mother or fetus.

Amnioinfusion

Intrapartum

Amnioinfusion involves the injection of sterile fluid into the uterine cavity, most commonly through the cervix using gravity flow or an infusion pump. Studies of patients with oligohydramnios in labour have demonstrated increased amniotic fluid index, decreased incidence of variable fetal heart rate decelerations and caesarean sections for fetal distress, and increased umbilical cord blood pH (Nageotte *et al* 1985, Lameier & Katz 1993). Amnioinfusion may be especially useful in patients with thick meconium, because it may reduce the incidence of fetal distress, emergency caesarean section and meconium aspiration (Macri *et al* 1992).

Prelabour amniorrhexis

In patients with preterm prelabour amniorrhexis, a modification of the traditional technique of amnioinfusion has been reported (Ogita *et al* 1988a). An indwelling catheter is introduced through the cervix and is held in position by two inflatable balloons and by the insertion of a cervical suture. The catheter also has channels for infusion of substances and sampling of amniotic fluid.

A preliminary study in 64 patients reported that a single daily dose of antibiotic, such as latamoxef sodium, cefoperazone sodium and cefotaxime sodium, was sufficient to provide therapeutic levels in the amniotic cavity for 24 hours (Ogita *et al* 1988a). In a study of 84 pregnancies with preterm prelabour amniorrhexis at less than 33 weeks of gestation, amnioinfusion of antibiotics, together with antiseptic washes of the upper vagina, was associated with a ten-fold reduction in the incidence of positive amniotic fluid cultures at delivery compared to the incidence on admission (from 40% to 4%) (Ogita *et al* 1988b). More widespread application of this form of treatment awaits confirmation of the results by other studies.

ANTIBIOTIC THERAPY

Preterm labour with intact membranes

Randomised trials on the use of antibiotic therapy in preterm labour with intact membranes have shown no beneficial effect in terms of the incidence of chorioamnionitis, endometritis or neonatal sepsis but in some of the studies there was a significant prolongation of the latency period (Table 4.2). In those studies that demonstrated significant prolongation of pregnancy, the mean length of time gained in utero was approximately 10 days.

Table 4.2. Randomised studies examining the effect of antibiotics on the incidence of preterm delivery in pregnancies with preterm labour and intact membranes.

Author	Antibiotic	N	Preterm delivery	
			Antibiotics	Controls
McGregor *et al* 1986	Erythromycin	17	13%	67%*
Newton *et al* 1989	Ampicillin / Erythromycin	96	38%	44%
Morales *et al* 1988	Ampicillin / Erythromycin	150	62%	85%*
Winkler *et al* 1988	Erythromycin	40	-	-
Newton *et al* 1991	Ampicillin	86	54%	63%
McGregor *et al* 1991a	Clindamycin	103	62%	62%
Romero *et al* 1993	Ampicillin / Erythromycin	277	53%	51%
Norman *et al* 1994	Ampicillin/ Metronidazole	81	-	-
Total	-	**850**	**53%**	**60%**

* $P < 0.05$

Preterm prelabour amniorrhexis

In preterm prelabour amniorrhexis, the aims of antibiotic therapy are (i) to eradicate occult infection, thereby reducing infectious complications for the mother and fetus, and (ii) to interrupt activation of those mechanisms that lead to preterm labour. Although antibiotic therapy is also aimed at reducing the risk of ascending infection, this is probably unnecessary because, as shown in Chapter 2, in patients with negative amniotic fluid and fetal blood cultures at presentation, subsequent development of intrauterine infection is unlikely.

A potential danger of prophylactic antibiotic use in women with preterm prelabour amniorrhexis is development of resistant organisms. Although there are case reports of neonatal sepsis with resistant organisms following antibiotic therapy for preterm prelabour amniorrhexis, it is not certain whether the use of antibiotics was responsible (McDuffie *et al* 1993).

Several studies on the use of antibiotics, such as clindamycin, mezlocillin, ampicillin, cefoxitin, gentamicin, during labour for chorioamnionitis have demonstrated measurable levels in cord blood at delivery and placental membranes (Gilstrap *et al* 1988a). Studies employing amniocentesis in patients with preterm prelabour amniorrhexis have shown that standard intravenous dosing protocols result in therapeutic levels of cefuroxime in maternal plasma, amniotic fluid and cord blood at delivery (DeLeeuw *et al* 1993).

Randomised studies

The studies assessing the value of antibiotic therapy in preterm prelabour amniorrhexis have not demonstrated a clear benefit on either the incidence of clinical chorioamnionitis or proven neonatal sepsis, but there was a small reduction in the incidence of endometritis (Table 4.3). This may be the consequence of the relatively small size of the populations examined and also the 'dilutional' effect of including all patients with amniorrhexis rather than only those with evidence of infection. Nevertheless, the majority of studies have shown a significant prolongation of pregnancy in those receiving antibiotics. This is important since premature delivery is the major complication of preterm prelabour amniorrhexis. In addition, prolongation of the pregnancy by even 24 hours exposes the fetus to the beneficial effect of corticosteroids.

Intrapartum antibiotics

In women with clinical chorioamnionitis, the use of antibiotics during labour may have a more protective effect against neonatal sepsis compared to the administration of antibiotics immediately after clamping of the cord. In three randomised studies on a total of 575 patients with clinical chorioamnionitis, the incidence of neonatal sepsis was only 2% in those that received intrapartum antibiotics compared to 13% for those that were treated after delivery (Sperling *et al* 1987, Gilstrap *et al* 1988b, Gibbs *et al* 1988).

Table 4.3. Randomised studies on the effect of antibiotic therapy (see table below) in patients with preterm prelabour amniorrhexis. Comparisons between groups are given as the 95% confidence interval of the odds ratio. The latter indicates the degree by which an outcome in the treated group differed from that in the controls. Table 4.4 below gives the definitions of the interval to delivery used in the various studies and the percentage of patients in each group that had not delivered within the given interval.

Study	N	Chorioamnionitis	Endometritis	Neonatal sepsis
1. Dunlop *et al* 1986	48	0.67-1.99	-	0.82-24.20
2. Amon *et al* 1988	82	0.54-4.80	0.43-5.47	0.02- 0.85
3. Johnston *et al* 1990	85	0.07-0.60	0.15-0.89	0.22-17.90
4. McGregor *et al* 1991b	55	0.45-2.90	-	-
5. Christmas *et al* 1992	94	0.62-4.57	0.05-2.33	0.23-19.20
6. Mercer *et al* 1992	220	0.42-1.69	0.36-3.17	0.45- 2.18
7. Lockwood *et al* 1993	72	-	-	0.13- 3.00
8. Owen *et al* 1993	117	0.29-0.82	0.11-1.21	0.08- 1.35
9. Ernest *et al* 1994	144	0.07-0.75	0.05-3.26	-
Total	**917**	**0.54-1.06**	**0.38-0.96**	**0.42-1.11**

Table 4.4. Interval to delivery.

Author	Definition of interval to delivery	Antibiotics	Controls
2. Amon *et al* 1988	More than 2 days from randomisation	70%	44%
3. Johnson *et al* 1990	More than 6 days from randomisation	45%	18%
5. Christmas *et al* 1992	More than 6 days from admission	42%	15%
6. Mercer *et al* 1992	More than 6 days from randomisation	27%	18%
7. Lockwood *et al* 1993	Mean (days) from amniorrhexis	11	6
8. Owen *et al* 1993	Mean (days) from amniorrhexis	12	7
9. Ernest *et al* 1994	Mean (days) from amniorrhexis	4	3
4. McGregor *et al* 1991b	Median (days) from randomisation	8	2

Antibiotic regimes used in the above studies
1. Cephalexin (250 -500 mg orally qds) until delivery.
2. Ampicillin (1g IV qds) for 24 hrs and then (500mg orally qds) until delivery.
3. Mezlocillin (?dose IV) for 48 hrs and then ampicillin (? dose orally) until delivery.
4. Erythromycin (333mg orally tds) until delivery.
5. Ampicillin (2g IV qds) and gentamicin (90mg IV loading followed by 60mg IV tds) and clindamycin (900mg IV tds) for 24 hrs, followed by amoxycillin and clavulanic acid (500mg orally tds) for seven days.
6. Erythromycin (333mg orally tds) until delivery.
7. Piperacillin sodium (3g IV qds) for 72 hrs.
8. Ampicillin (1g IV qds) for 24hrs and then (500mg orally qds) until delivery.
9. Benzylpenicillin (1 million units IV 4 hrly) for 24 hrs and then phenoxy-methylpenicillin (250 mg orally bd) for 48 hrs.

STEROID THERAPY

Preterm labour with intact membranes

Randomised studies examining the effect of corticosteroids in pregnancies at risk of preterm delivery with intact membranes have demonstrated that the risks of neonatal death, respiratory distress syndrome and periventricular haemorrhage are approximately half in the treated group compared to the controls (Table 4.5).

Table 4.5. Randomised studies on the effect of maternal corticosteroids on fetal outcome in women with preterm labour and intact membranes. The last column reports the outcome measures examined in each study and the table below summarises the pooled odds ratios for each outcome.

Author	Gestation	N	Steroid	Outcome
Liggins & Howie 1972	<37 wks	1,135	Betamethasone	1,2,3
Block *et al* 1977	<37 wks	175	Betamethasone	1,3
Morrison *et al* 1978	<34 wks	196	Hydrocortisone	1,3
Papageorgiou *et al* 1979	<34 wks	146	Betamethasone	1,3
Schutte *et al* 1979	<32 wks	122	Betamethasone	1,3
Taeusch *et al* 1979	<34 wks	127	Dexamethasone	1,3
Doran *et al* 1980	<34 wks	144	Betamethasone	1,2,3
Teramo *et al* 1980	<36 wks	80	Betamethasone	1,3
Schmidt *et al* 1984	<34 wks	149	Hydrocortisone	1,3
Gamsu *et al* 1989	<34 wks	268	Betamethasone	1,2,3
Collaborative group 1981	<34 wks	757	Dexamethasone	1,3

Outcome studied	Pooled odds ratios (95% CI)
1. Respiratory distress syndrome	0.48 (0.40-0.58)
2. Periventricular haemorrhage	0.44 (0.22-0.88)
3. Early neonatal death	0.59 (0.47-0.75)

Preterm prelabour amniorrhexis

In pregnancies with amniorrhexis there is a potential risk that steroid therapy may suppress inflammatory and immune responses leading to a higher likelihood of infection.

There are six randomised studies which have specifically investigated the effect of maternal corticosteroid administration in pregnancies with preterm prelabour amniorrhexis involving a total of 751 pregnancies (Table 4.6).

Table 4.6. Randomised studies on the effect of maternal corticosteroids on maternal and fetal outcome in women with preterm prelabour amniorrhexis at less than 34 weeks. The last column reports the outcome measures examined in each study and the table below summarises the pooled odds ratios for each outcome.

Author	N	Steroid	Outcome
Garite *et al* 1981	159	Betamethasone	1,2,5
Schmidt *et al* 1984	41	Hydrocortisone	5
Iams *et al* 1985	73	Betamethasone	1,2,4,5,6
Nelson *et al* 1985	68	Betamethasone	1,4,5,6
Morales *et al* 1986a	245	Dexamethasone	1,3,4,5,6
Morales *et al* 1989	165	Betamethasone	1,3,4,5,6

Outcome studied	Pooled odds ratios (95% CI)
1. Clinical chorioamnionitis	0.73 (0.48-1.10)
2. Maternal endometritis	2.97 (1.43-6.18)
3. Intraventricular haemorrhage	0.51 (0.26-0.99)
4. Perinatal mortality	0.65 (0.36-1.17)
5. Respiratory distress syndrome	0.45 (0.33-0.62)
6. Neonatal sepsis	1.22 (0.56-2.62)

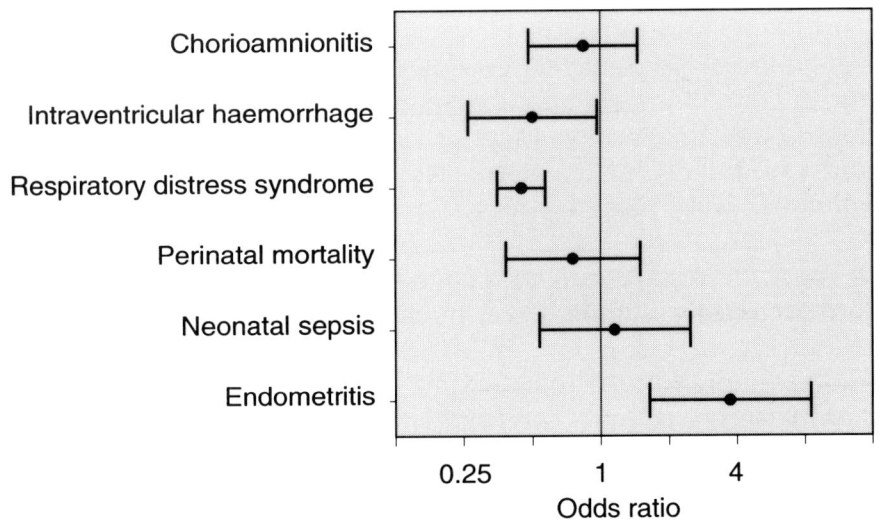

The data of these studies have demonstrated that, as with preterm labour and intact membranes, in preterm prelabour amniorrhexis the use of corticosteroids compared to controls is associated with approximately half as much risk of neonatal death, respiratory distress syndrome and intraventricular haemorrhage.

The beneficial effects of steroids are not accompanied by increased risk of neonatal sepsis or clinical chorioamnionitis, although there is a small but significant increase in risk for postpartum endometritis.

TOCOLYTIC THERAPY

Tocolytic therapy is aimed at stopping or reducing the contractility of the uterus, thereby reducing the incidence of preterm delivery. Many agents have been studied, including betamimetics, inhibitors of prostaglandin synthesis, calcium channel blocking drugs, relaxin, alcohol, progestagens, nitrates and even acupuncture.

The most commonly used agents are betamimetics, such as salbutamol or ritodrine. These are thought to act both as agonists of myometrial receptors, causing reduced intracellular calcium and consequent myometrial relaxation, and as antagonists of amniotic membrane receptors, thereby reducing prostaglandin production (Collins *et al* 1993). Prostaglandin synthesis inhibitors act to reduce the amount of prostaglandin produced by the membranes and hence to less stimulation of the uterus. Calcium channel blockers of the dihydropyridine group, such as nifedipine, reduce the intracellular concentration of calcium leading to myometrial relaxation. Magnesium sulphate may also act to reduce intracellular calcium. Nitrates are thought to act by donation of nitric oxide, which is a potent smooth muscle relaxant.

All tocolytic agents are associated with adverse effects ranging from tachycardia, chest pain, hyperglycaemia, hypokalaemia and pulmonary oedema with beta agonists, bronchospasm, gastric irritation, premature closure of the ductus arteriosus and oligohydramnios with prostaglandin synthesis inhibitors, and flushing, palpitations, diplopia and respiratory depression with magnesium sulphate (ABPI Data Sheet Compendium 1994, British National Formulary 1994).

Preterm labour with intact membranes

Randomised, placebo controlled trials have demonstrated that in preterm labour with intact membranes both beta agonists and prostaglandin synthesis inhibitors can reduce the proportion of deliveries which occur within 24 hours from the onset of labour (Table 4.7).

Consequently tocolytics are beneficial in maximising the effect of corticosteroids. Their effect in reducing the incidence of preterm delivery is less marked.

Table 4.7. Randomised trials examining the effect of beta agonists on prolongation of pregnancy in patients with preterm labour and intact membranes.

Author	N	Delivery within 24 hours	
		Tocolysis	**Controls**
Ingemarsson 1976	30	0%	67%*
Spellacy *et al* 1979	29	43%	73%
Larsen *et al* 1980	176	8%	13%
Christensen *et al* 1980	30	0%	38%*
Howard *et al* 1982	33	13%	11%
Cotton *et al* 1984	38	32%	58%
Larsen *et al* 1986	99	10%	32%*
Leveno *et al* 1986	106	28%	48%*
Calder & Patel 1985	76	11%	23%
Total	**617**	**27%**	**33%***

* $P < 0.05$

Preterm prelabour amniorrhexis

In preterm labour after prelabour amniorrhexis there is reluctance to give tocolytics because amniorrhexis is often associated with infection and there are theoretical worries that tocolytic use may contain a fetus within an infected uterine environment. Additionally, the side effects of the tocolytic agents themselves, such as tachycardia, may mask signs of maternal infection.

Prophylactic tocolysis

Two randomised studies on a total of 90 patients with preterm prelabour amniorrhexis and no evidence of clinical infection at 25-36 weeks of gestation reported that the proportion of women remaining undelivered 10 days after amniorrhexis was not significantly higher in those receiving oral prophylactic tocolysis (24%), compared to those receiving placebo (18%; Levy & Warsof 1985, Dunlop *et al* 1986).

Therapeutic tocolysis

Two randomised studies on a total of 109 women with preterm labour after prelabour amniorrhexis reported that the use of intravenous tocolysis was not associated with a significantly higher proportion of women that had not delivered within one week after the onset of labour (Table 4.8; Christensen *et al* 1980, Garite *et al* 1987).

Weiner *et al* (1988) examined the use of tocolysis in 109 women with preterm labour following prelabour amniorrhexis at less than 34 weeks gestation; although tocolysis was not associated with prolongation of pregnancy in the total group, in the subgroup with preterm labour at less than 28 weeks, the average interval from onset of contractions to delivery was 232 hours for the tocolytic group compared to 53 hours for the placebo group.

Table 4.8. Studies investigating the use of tocolytic agents in preterm labour after prelabour amniorrhexis.

Author	N	Delivery within seven days	
		Tocolysis	**Controls**
Christensen *et al* 1980	30	79%	94%
Garite *et al* 1987	79	69%	68%
Weiner *et al* 1988	109	NS*	NS

* In this study there was no significant difference between the groups but percentages were not provided

These results suggest that, in preterm labour following preterm prelabour amniorrhexis, the effectiveness of tocolysis is dependent on gestational age. Other factors that may influence the efficacy of tocolysis are the amount of residual amniotic fluid and the presence of infection.

Silver *et al* (1989) studied 70 singleton pregnancies with preterm prelabour amniorrhexis at 25-34 weeks of gestation and reported an inverse relationship between the amniotic fluid index and the likelihood of successful tocolysis; only 8% of the group with oligohydramnios were undelivered at one week compared to 57% in the group with adequate amniotic fluid volume throughout.

Another study of 86 women in preterm labour, who had amniotic fluid sampled and were commenced on tocolytic treatment, reported that tocolysis was successful in only 7% of those with evidence of intrauterine infection compared to 93% for those without infection (Cherouny *et al* 1992).

DELIVERY

Abdominal or vaginal

There is controversy over the optimal type of delivery for the preterm infant. The advocates of caesarean section argue that, because preterm infants have a soft skull, vaginal delivery may cause birth trauma. In contrast, caesarean delivery is associated with increased risk for the mother, particularly if the lower segment is not well formed and a classical incision is needed.

Retrospective studies and anecdotal reports tend to prejudice the obstetrician towards vaginal or caesarean delivery, making it almost impossible to perform randomised trials. A recent survey in the United Kingdom reported that, in patients with uncomplicated preterm labour, 76% of obstetricians advocated routine caesarean section for breech presentation; the respective percentage for cephalic presentation was 12% (Penn & Steer 1991).

Furthermore, potential benefit to the fetus must be weighed against the increased risk of perioperative maternal complications, particularly if the lower segment is not well formed and a classical incision is needed. For instance, Lao *et al* (1993) compared maternal blood loss between patients who had classical caesarean section

(CCS) and lower segment caesarean section (LSCS) at 34 weeks gestation or less. Sixty-two women were compared after matching for gestational age at delivery, the type of anaesthesia, and the prior use of tocolytic therapy and there was a significantly greater incidence of severe bleeding (>1,000 mL) at operation in those that had a classical as compared to a lower segment, caesarean section.

Cephalic presentation

Several retrospective studies have reported that for preterm infants in cephalic presentation there is no significant improvement in survival for those delivered by caesarean section compared to those delivered vaginally (Table 4.9). Malloy *et al* (1989) reported that, after correction for maternal demographic characteristics, there is no significant relationship between the method of delivery and survival. Similarly, in the study of Amon *et al* (1987), although overall survival was higher in those delivered by caesarean section, when gestational age and birth weight were adjusted for, there was no significant difference in outcome between the abdominal and vaginal delivery groups. In the study of Kitchen *et al* (1985) the incidence of intraventricular haemorrhage was also examined and this was not significantly different in those delivered vaginally (45%) compared to those delivered abdominallly (33%).

Table 4.9. Retrospective studies reporting on survival by mode of preterm delivery in pregnancies with cephalic presentation.

Author	Criteria	N	Survival	
			Vaginal	**Abdominal**
Kitchen *et al* 1985	24-28 weeks	326	51%	63%
Olshan *et al* 1984	700-1,500 g	248	66%	78%
Amon *et al* 1987	< 1,000 g	476	31%	49%
Malloy *et al* 1989	500-1,500 g	3,095	NS	NS

NS This study reported no significant difference between the groups but did not provide the percentages

Breech presentation

The incidence of breech presentation is about 40% at 20 weeks, 25% at 30 weeks and 3% at term (Sorensen *et al* 1979). Most studies examining the optimal mode of delivery for the preterm fetus presenting by the breech suggest that, for those with birth weight of less than 1,500 g, abdominal delivery may be associated with improved outcome (Table 4.10).

Table 4.10. Studies examining neonatal survival and incidence of intraventricular haemorrhage (IVH) in preterm infants presenting by the breech, according to route of delivery (Vag = vaginal, CS = caesarean section).

Author	Criteria	N	Survival		IVH	
			Vag	CS	Vag	CS
Kauppila 1975	<2500 g	326	67%	67%	-	-
Bowes 1977	500-1499 g	49	38%	76%	-	-
Goldenberg & Nelson 1977	<2500 g	274	57%	85%	-	-
Lyons & Papsin 1978	<2500 g	47	84%	89%	-	-
Ingemarsson *et al* 1978	<37 wks	90	85%	95%	-	-
Karp *et al* 1979	1000-2500 g	54	79%	80%	-	-
Mann & Gallant 1979	<2000 g	102	53%	67%	-	-
Duenhoelter *et al* 1979	1000-2499 g	88	84%	98%	11%	0%
Woods 1979	1000-2499 g	87	75%	86%	-	-
Kauppila *et al* 1981	1000-2499 g	434	92%	98%	-	-
Geirsson *et al* 1982	<37 wks	38	41%	100%	-	-
Main *et al* 1983	750-1499 g	216	42%	71%	46%	34%
Effer *et al* 1983	500-1499 g	93	55%	67%	-	-
Lamont *et al* 1983	<1500 g	31	63%	100%	59%	22%
Rosen & Chik 1984	<2500 g	223	69%	93%	-	-
Doyle *et al* 1985	501-1499 g	131	52%	85%	29%	13%
Morales & Koerten 1986	500-1500 g	148	74%	91%	57%	27%
Malhotra *et al* 1994	28-36 wks	224	64%	82%	-	-
Total		**2,655**	**68%**	**84%**	**41%**	**22%**

However, the studies are either retrospective reviews or poorly controlled trials. Consequently it is possible that, at least in part, the better results associated with abdominal delivery were due to selection bias, because in those cases thought to carry a poor prognosis, obstetricians may have been reluctant to subject the mother to the potential complications of caesarean section. For example, in a study of 843 breech deliveries, although the perinatal mortality was lower in those delivered abdominally (10%), compared to the vaginal delivery group (23%), the birth weights of the latter were significantly lower (Brown *et al* 1994). Similarly, in a retrospective analysis of 224 breech deliveries at 28-36 weeks gestation, although the combined intrapartum and neonatal mortality was significantly higher in those delivered vaginally (36%) rather than abdominally (18%), there was no significant difference when the data were adjusted for gestation at delivery or birth weight (Malhotra *et al* 1994).

Additionally, retrospective studies comparing their recent results, when the incidence of caesarean section is much higher, with those of historical controls, may overestimate the contribution of the mode of delivery to improved survival, which, in reality, may be mainly due to improved neonatal care. For example, Dietl *et al* (1991) reported that, for infants delivered before 32 weeks of gestation or weighing less than 1,500 g, in their hospital, the caesarean section rate had increased from 28% in 1977-1982 to 87% in 1982-1987; during this period survival had increased from 63% to 70%. In a recent study on 899 liveborn singleton non-malformed infants born at less than 32 weeks gestation, logistic regression analysis was performed and demonstrated that breech presenting infants had a significantly lower mortality risk when born by caesarean section compared with vaginal delivery (Gravenhorst *et al* 1993).

The incidence of intracranial haemorrhage also appears to be lower in the abdominal delivery group than in infants delivered vaginally (Table 4.10). In another study of 189 infants with birth weight of less than 1,000 g, routine neonatal brain ultrasound scans demonstrated that both the incidence and severity of periventricular / intraventricular haemorrhage were higher in those delivered vaginally (52%) than in those delivered abdominally (25%; Philip & Allan 1991). However, abdominal delivery may not be protective against the development of brain haemorrhage if the caesarean section is performed after the onset of labour. Thus, in a study of 89 infants weighing less than 1,750 g, ultrasound examination within one hour of delivery demonstrated germinal layer /intraventricular haemorrhage in 32% of the cases, and the incidence and severity of haemorrhage were higher in those born after labour regardless of the subsequent route of delivery (Anderson *et al* 1988).

Elective episiotomy

In a study of 42 infants with birth weights of 751-1,250 g that were delivered vaginally by the vertex, outcome was examined in relation to whether the infants were delivered by obstetricians who practised routine episiotomy or by those that performed episiotomies only if absolutely necessary (Lobb *et al* 1986). There were no significant differences in survival or the incidence of periventricular haemorrhage between the two groups.

Elective use of forceps

There is no evidence that the elective use of obstetrics forceps for delivery of the preterm infant is beneficial.

A study examining factors related to the development of intraventricular haemorrhage in 70 infants, delivered vaginally and weighing 800-1,350 g, reported that the incidence of haemorrhage was 22% in those that delivered spontaneously and 43% in those delivered by forceps (Haesslein *et al* 1979).

In another study of 1,065 infants with birth weight of 1,000-2,500 g that were delivered vaginally with a vertex presentation, the rate of neonatal death in the 394 delivered by low forceps was not significantly different from that in the 671 who delivered spontaneously (spontaneous 148/1000 versus forceps 35/1000 for birth weight 1,000-1,500 g, 42/1000 versus 13/1000 for birth weight 1,501-2,000 g and 8/1000 versus 7/1000 for birth weight 1,501-2,000 g) (Schwartz *et al* 1983).

In a randomised study investigating the elective use of forceps in 46 infants delivered vaginally at 28-35 weeks of gestation, the use of forceps was not associated with a significant reduction in the incidence of retinal haemorrhages, a marker of cranial trauma which occurred in 6% of the total group (Maltau *et al* 1984).

Intrapartum fetal heart rate patterns

A study, comparing fetal heart rate patterns in labour at 28-35 weeks of gestation in 267 pregnancies complicated by prelabour amniorrhexis with those in 130 cases with preterm labour and intact membranes, reported that the incidence of caesarean section for fetal distress was 8% for the group with amniorrhexis compared to 2% for the group with intact membranes; in more than 75% of the cases of fetal distress associated with amniorrhexis, the heart rate patterns were consistent with umbilical cord compression, most probably due to the associated oligohydramnios (Moberg *et al* 1984).

PULMONARY HYPOPLASIA

Pathophysiology of pulmonary hypoplasia

Suggested mechanisms for the causes of pulmonary hypoplasia in oligohydramnios include extrinsic compression of the fetal lungs, enhanced outflow of fetal lung fluid, and cessation of fetal breathing movements (Lawrence and Rosenfeld 1986).

In the absence of amniotic fluid, the fetal thorax and consequently the lungs are subjected to extrinsic compression which interferes with normal development. This concept of fetal compression is supported by other sequelae of oligohydramnios such as talipes and Potter's facies.

In animal studies, iatrogenic oligohydramnios, by occlusion of the fetal bladder neck or by chronic shunting of amniotic fluid into the maternal abdominal cavity, was associated with the development of pulmonary hypoplasia (Nakayama *et al* 1983). When fetal thoracic compression was relieved, in the bladder-outlet occlusion group, by constant intra-amniotic infusion of saline until term, the neonates had nearly normal-sized lungs. Further evidence for the association between lung compression and pulmonary hypoplasia was provided by the demonstration that in fetal sheep placement of inflated balloons in the pleural cavity resulted in pulmonary hypoplasia (Harrison *et al* 1980). Chronic tracheal drainage in fetal sheep resulted in pulmonary hypoplasia (Alcorn *et al* 1977). In the human, excessive loss of lung fluid could be the consequence of extrinsic compression of the fetal thorax or an increase in the alveolar-amniotic pressure gradient. Supportive evidence for the latter was provided by the demonstration that in amniorrhexis the intra-amniotic pressure is reduced (Nicolini *et al* 1989).

Fetal breathing movements may be important for normal lung growth and their cessation could cause pulmonary hypoplasia. This has been shown in animal studies where transection of the cervical spinal cord and consequent interruption of breathing movements resulted in pulmonary hypoplasia (Wigglesworth *et al* 1977, Wigglesworth & Desai 1979, Liggins *et al* 1981). In the human, it was postulated that failure of lung growth in association with oligohydramnios could be due to inhibition of fetal breathing movements (Wigglesworth *et al* 1981). However, the mechanisms by which oligohydramnios might reduce fetal breathing movements is obscure. Extrinsic compression of the thorax may not be the explanation because fetal breathing is almost exclusively diaphragmatic in type and the chest wall plays a passive role (Poore & Walker 1980). It has also been suggested that uterine contractions may inhibit fetal breathing by elevating prostaglandin levels, which are known to abolish fetal breathing movements in labour (Blott *et al* 1990).

Diagnosis of pulmonary hypoplasia

The conflicting results on the value of antenatal tests in the prediction of pulmonary hypoplasia (see below) could be the consequence of the different criteria used for the diagnosis of pulmonary hypoplasia. These include (i) postmortem evidence of low lung DNA content or low lung to body weight ratio or reduced radial alveolar count, or chest radiographs demonstrating small-volume lungs, (ii) clinical evidence of high peak inspiratory pressures (in excess of 30 cm of water) during positive pressure ventilation, both for resuscitation and during subsequent respiratory support (Moessinger *et al* 1987, Blott *et al* 1990, Ohlsson *et al* 1991).

Antenatal prediction of pulmonary hypoplasia

Attempts at antenatal prediction of pulmonary hypoplasia have focused on assessment of lung size, amniotic fluid volume and fetal breathing movements. Several studies have attempted to determine fetal lung size by ultrasonography in pregnancies with preterm prelabour amniorrhexis and they reported favourable results in the prediction of pulmonary hypoplasia (Table 4.11).

In contrast to fetal lung size, the studies that attempted to quantify the degree of oligohydramnios have generally reported poor prediction of pulmonary hypoplasia (Table 4.12, Figure 4.1).

A possible explanation is that amniotic fluid volume in prelabour amniorrhexis varies considerably on a daily basis, decreasing by as much as 75% and increasing by up to 200% from one day to the next (Harding *et al* 1991).

Table 4.11. True positive rate (TP) and false positive rate (FP) of reduced fetal lung size in the prediction of pulmonary hypoplasia (PH) in cases of preterm prelabour amniorrhexis. Reduction in lung size had been defined as measurement below the 2.5th centile of the appropriate normal range.

Author	N	PH	Lung size	TP	FP
D'Alton *et al* 1992	16	6	External thoracic to abdominal circumference ratio	100%	0%
Roberts & Mitchell 1990	20	12	External thoracic circumference	66%	0%
Blott *et al* 1990	20	5	Internal thoracic circumference	60%	6%
Blott *et al* 1990	20	5	Lung area	60%	13%
Roberts & Mitchell 1990	20	12	Lung length	92%	0%

Table 4.12. True positive rate (TP) and false positive rate (FP) of reduced amniotic fluid volume in the prediction of pulmonary hypoplasia (PH) in cases of preterm prelabour amniorrhexis. Amniotic fluid volume was measured as amniotic fluid index (AFI), or vertical diameter (VD) of amniotic fluid pockets.

Author	N	PH	Amniotic fluid volume	TP	FP
Roberts & Mitchell 1990	20	12	Mean VD of largest pool for all examinations <1.5cm	100%	50%
Rotschild *et al* 1990	88	14	VD of largest pool <1 cm	50%	35%
Rotschild *et al* 1990	88	14	VD of largest pool ≤2 cm	36%	27%
Vergani *et al* 1994	63	15	Median VD of all pools ≤2cm	100%	62%
Ohlsson *et al* 1991	23	3	AFI ≤5 cm	100%	60%
Carroll *et al* 1995a	108	6	AFI ≤5 cm	100%	28%

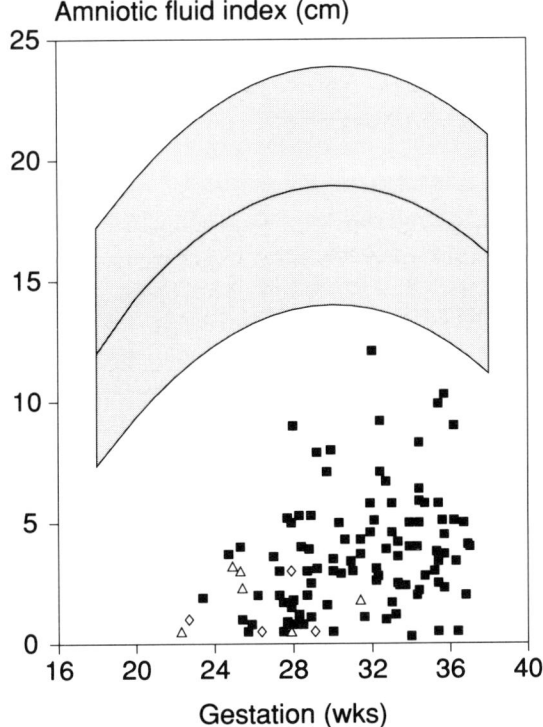

Figure 4.1. Amniotic fluid index in 89 patients with preterm prelabour amniorrhexis plotted on the normal range for gestation (shaded area, mean ± 2 SDs). (■)= survivors, (△)= deaths due to complications of prematurity, (◊)= deaths due to pulmonary hypoplasia. Adapted from Carroll *et al* 1995a.

Studies evaluating fetal breathing movements in the prediction of impaired lung growth reported conflicting results (Table 4.13).

Table 4.13. True positive rate (TP) and false positive rate (FP) of absent fetal breathing movements in the prediction of pulmonary hypoplasia (PH) in cases of preterm prelabour amniorrhexis.

Author	N	PH	TP	FP
Fox & Moessinger 1985	7	3	0%	0%
Moessinger *et al* 1987	14	9	0%	0%
Blott *et al* 1990	20	5	100%	0%
Ohlsson *et al* 1991	23	3	33%	30%
Carroll *et al* 1995a	108	6	67%	37%
Total	**172**	**26**	**58%**	**18%**

A possible explanation is the different definitions for presence of breathing activity used in the various studies. Blott *et al* (1990) considered breathing to be present if at least one thoracic movement occurred every six seconds for at least one minute. Moessinger *et al* (1987) defined breathing movements by the presence of three breaths in a period of six seconds. Ohlsson *et al* (1991) defined the presence of fetal breathing as breathing movements that lasted for more than six seconds with a breath-to-breath interval of at least six seconds. The discrepancy in results may also be the consequence of differences in the gestational age of patients studied, since fetal breathing activity is known to change with gestation (Fox *et al* 1979).

Doppler assessment

Blood flow in the ductus arteriosus, as assessed by Doppler ultrasound, is altered by breathing movements. In a study of 12 cases of preterm prelabour amniorrhexis and severe oligohydramnios, the alteration in ductal blood flow by breathing movements was normal in seven cases with normal lungs, and reduced in all five cases with pulmonary hypoplasia (Van Eyck *et al* 1990). The validity of these findings requires further study.

RECOMMENDED MANAGEMENT

Initial assessment

In patients with suspected amniorrhexis the diagnosis may be confirmed by performing a sterile speculum examination and testing the fluid with a Nitrazine indicator. Digital cervico-vaginal examination should be avoided. The value of cervico-vaginal swabs for culture is uncertain.

Ultrasound examination should be performed to exclude fetal defects, to estimate fetal weight and to determine the presentation.

An amniocentesis, and also cordocentesis in centres with the appropriate experience, is essential for the diagnosis/exclusion of subclinical infection. The Gram stain and leukocyte count will provide an early (within one hour) indication of possible infection but this requires confirmation by culture, which provides results within two days.

Management of patients with negative cultures

In this group, subsequent development of infection is unlikely and there is no need for hospitalisation or bed rest.

>34 weeks

These patients are best managed expectantly, awaiting spontaneous vaginal delivery. There is no need for antibiotics, steroids or tocolytics.

24-34 weeks

In this group, the main risk is that of prematurity and therefore, the aim is to prolong the pregnancy.

Corticosteroids are of proven value and should be given. There is no evidence that the use of prophylactic antibiotics is beneficial. If labour starts, tocolytics should be administered and for breech presentation, if the gestation is less than 32 weeks or the estimated fetal weight less than 1,500 g, delivery by caesarean section may be preferable to vaginal delivery. If the latter is chosen, there is no evidence in favour of elective episiotomy or use of forceps.

<24 weeks

In this group the main risks are those of miscarriage / preterm delivery and pulmonary hypoplasia.

Termination of the pregnancy should be one of the options to be discussed with the parents. In those that continue with the pregnancy, the value of chronic amnioinfusion in reducing the incidence of pulmonary hypoplasia requires further investigation. If the pregnancy continues to beyond 24 weeks, management is as above.

Management of patients with positive cultures

This group will go into spontaneous labour within a few days of amniorrhexis. The main risks to the baby are those of prematurity and sepsis. Additionally, the mother is at risk of infectious complications. These patients should be hospitalised and receive appropriate antibiotic therapy.

>34 weeks

This group is best managed by induction of labour and intrapartum administration of antibiotics.

24-34 weeks

These patients are best managed expectantly. The use of corticosteroids is beneficial and there is no associated increase in risk of clinical chorioamnionitis or neonatal sepsis. Antibiotics should be administered, but the optimal regime and effectiveness need to be assessed by further studies. If labour starts, tocolytics should not be given and if the presentation is breech, caesarean section may be preferable to vaginal delivery.

<24 weeks

In this group the main risk is progression to miscarriage or preterm delivery of a septic infant. Management options to be discussed with the parents include termination of the pregnancy or aggressive attempts to prevent early delivery including maternal antibiotic therapy, and, in addition, possible amnioinfusion with antimicrobial agents.

Preterm Prelabour Amniorrhexis:
Management Protocol 1995

NO INFECTION		INFECTION
Expectant management -Spontaneous delivery	**>34 weeks**	**Labour induction** -Intrapartum antibiotics
Expectant management -Corticosteroids -Therapeutic tocolysis	**24-34 weeks**	**Expectant management** -Corticosteroids -Antibiotics
Expectant management -Amnioinfusion **or** **Termination of pregnancy**	**<24 weeks**	**Expectant management** -Antibiotics -Amnioinfusion **or** **Termination of pregnancy**

REFERENCES

Abe T. The detection of rupture of the fetal membranes with the nitrazine indicator. Am J Obstet Gynecol 1940;39:400-4.

ABPI Data Sheet Compendium. Association of the British Pharmaceutical Industry.1994.

Alcorn D, Adamson TM, Lambert TF, Maloney JE, Ritchie BC, Robinson PM. Morphological effects of of trachal ligation and drainage in the fetal lamb lung. J Anat 1977;123:649-66.

Amon E, Lewis SV, Sibai BM, Villar MA, Arheart KL. Ampicillin prophylaxis in preterm premature rupture of the membranes:a prospective randomised study. Am J Obstet Gynecol 1988;159:539-43.

Amon E, Sibai BN, Anderson GD, Mabie WC. Obstetric variables predicting survival of the immature newborn (<1000 g): A five year experiece at a single centre. Obstet Gynecol 1987;156:1380-9.

Anderson GD, Bada HS, Sibai BM, Harvey C, Korones SB, Magill HL, Wong SP, Tullis K. The relationship between labour and route of delivery in the preterm infant. Am J Obstet Gynecol 1988;158:1382-90.

Averette HE, Hopman BC, Ferguson JH. Cytodiagnosis of ruptured fetal membranes. Am J Obstet Gynecol 1963;87:226-35.

Baptisti A. Chemical test for the determination of ruptured membranes. Am J Obstet Gynecol 1938;35:688-90.

Baumgarten K, Moser S. The technique of fibrin adhesion for premature rupture of the membranes during pregnancy. J Perinat Med 1986;14:43-7.

Berlind MW. Test for rupotured bag of waters. Am J Obstet Gynecol 1932;24: 918-20.

Block MF, Kling OR, Crosby WM. Antenatal glucocorticoid therapy for the prevention of respiratory distress syndrome in the premature infant. Obstet Gynecol 1977;50:186-90.

Blott M, Greenough A, Nicolaides KH, Campbell S. The ultrasonographic assessment of the fetal thorax and fetal breathing movements in the prediction of pulmonary hypoplasia. Early Hum Devel 1990;21:143-51.

Bowes WA. Results of the intensive perinatal management of very low birthweight infants. In: Preterm labour.Proceedings of the Fifth stufy group of the Royal College of Obstetricians and Gynaecologists.p 331-55. Ed Anderson A.RCOG London. 1977.

British National Formulary. British Medical Association / Royal Pharmaceutical Society of Great Britain (1994).

Brosens I, Gordon H. The cytologic diagnosis of ruptured membranes using Nile Blue sulfate staining. J Obstet Gynecol Br Commonwealth 1965;72:342-6.

Brown CL, Ludwiczak MH, Blanco JD, Hirsch CE. Cervical dilatation: accuracy of visual and digital examinations. Obstet Gynecol 1993;81;215-16.

Brown L, Karrison T, Cibils LA. Mode of delivery and perinatal results in breech presentation. Am J Obstet Gynecol 1994;171:28-34.

Calder AA, Patel NB. Are betamimetics worthwhile in preterm labour? In: Preterm labour and its consequences. Proceedings of the thirteenth study group of the Royal College of Obstetricians and Gynaecologists.p 209-18. Ed Beard RW. RCOG. London.1985.

Campbell BA, Newman RB, Stramm SL. Uterine activity after premature rupture of the membranes. Am J Obstet Gynecol 1991;165:422-5.

Carlan SJ, O'Brien WF, Parsons MT, Lense JJ. Preterm premature rupture of membranes: A randomised study of home versus hospital management. Obstet Gynecol 1993;81:61-4.

Carroll SG, Blott M, Nicolaides KH. Preterm prelabour amniorrhexis: outcome of livebirths. Obstet Gynecol 1995 (In press).

Chalmers I, Enkin M, Keirse MJNC. In: Effective care in pregnancy and childbirth. Oxford University Press. England. 1992.

Cherouny PH, Pankuch GA, Botti JJ, Appelbaum PC. The presence of amniotic fluid leukoattractants accurately identifies histologic chorioamnionitis and predicts tocolytic efficacy in patients with idiopathic preterm labour. Am J Obstet Gynecol 1992;167:683-8.

Christensen KK, Ingemarsson I, Leideman T, Solum H, Svenningsen N. Effect of ritodrine on labour after premature rupture of the membranes. Obstet Gynecol 1980;55:187-90.

Christmas JT, Cox SM, Andrews W, Dax J, Leveno KJ, Gilstrap LC. Expectant management of preterm ruptured membranes:effects of antimicrobial therapy. Obstet Gynecol 1992;80:759-62.

Collaborative group on antenatal steroid therapy. Effect of antenatal dexamethasone therapy on prevention of respiratory distress syndrome. Am J Obstet Gynecol 1981;141:276-87.

Collins PL, Zink E, Moore RM, Roberts JM, Maguire ME, Moore JJ. Ritodrine: A beta adrenergic receptor antagonist in human amnion. Am J Obstet Gynecol 1993;168:143-51.

Cotton DB, Strassner HT, Hill LM, Schifrin BS, Paul RH. Comparison of magnesium sulfate, terbutaline and a placebo for inhibition of preterm labour. A randomised study. J Reprod Med 1984;29:92-7.

D'Alton M, Mercer B, Riddick E, Dudley D. Serial thoracic versus abdominal circumference ratios for the prediction of pulmonary hypoplasia in premature rupture of the membranes remote from term. Am J Obstet Gynecol 1992;166:658-63.

DeLeeuw J, Roumen FJME, Bouckaert PXJM, Cremers HMHG, Vree TB. Achievement of therapeutic concentrations of cefuroxime in early preterm gestations with premature rupture of the membranes. Obstet Gynecol 1993;81:255-60.

Dietl J, Arnold H, Haas G, Mentzel H, Pietsch Breitfeld-B, Hirsch HA. Delivery of very premature infants: does the caesarean section rate relate to mortality, morbidity, or long-term outcome? Arch Gynecol Obstet 1991;249: 191-200.

Doran TA, Swyer P, MacMurray B, Mahon W, Enhorning G, Bernstein A, Falk M, Wood M. Results of a double blind controlled study on the use of betamethasone in the prevention of respiratory distress syndrome. Am J Obstet Gynecol 1980;136:313-20.

Doyle LW, Rickards AL, Ford GW, Pepperell RJ, Kitchen W. Outcome for the very low birth weight (501-1499 g) singleton breech: Benefit of casarean section. Aust NZ J Obstet Gynecol 1985;25:259-65.

Duenhoelter JH, Wells E, Reisch JS, Santos-Ramos R, Jiminez JM. A paired controlled study of vaginal and abdominal delivery of the low birth weight breech fetus. Obstet Gynecol 1979;54:310-13.

Dunlop PDM, Crowley PA, Lamont RF, Hawkins DF. Preterm ruptured membranes, no contractions. J Obstet Gynecol 1986;7:92-6.

Effer SB, Saigal S, Rand C, Hunter DJS, Stoskopf B, Harper AC, Nimrod C, Milner R. Effect of delivery method on outcomes in the very low birth weight breech infant: Is the improved survival related to cesarean section or other perinatal care maneuvres? Am J Obstet Gynecol 1983;145:123-8.

Eriksen NL, Parisi VM, Daust S, Flamm B, Garite TJ, Cox SM. Fetal fibronectin: A method for detecting the presence of amniotic fluid. Obstet Gynecol 1992;80:451-4.

Ernest JM, Givner LB. A prospective, randomised, placebo-contolled trial of penicillin in preterm premature rupture of membranes. Am J Obstet Gynecol 1994;170:516-21.

Fox HE, Inglis J, Steinbrecher M. Fetal breathing movements in uncomplicated pregnancies: Relationship to gestational age. Am J Obstet Gynecol 1979;134: 544-6.

Fox HE, Moessinger AC. Fetal breathing movements and lung hypoplasia: Preliminary human observations. Am J Obstet Gynecol 1985;151:531-3.

Friedman ML, McElin TW. Diagnosis of ruptured fetal membranes. Clinical study and review of the literature. Am J Obstet Gynecol 1969;104:544-50.

Gamsu HR, Mullinger BM, Donnai P, Dash CH. Antenatal administration of Betamethasone to prevent respiratory distress syndrome in preterm infants: report of a UK multicentre trial. Br J Obstet Gynaecol 1989;96:401-10.

Garite TJ, Freeman RK, Linzey EM, Braly PS, Dorchester WL. Prospective randomised study of corticosteroids in the management of premature rupture of the membranes and the premature gestation. Am J Obstet Gynecol 1981;141:508-14.

Garite TJ, Keegan KA, Freeman RK, Nageotte MP. A randomised trial of ritodrine tocolysis versus expectant management in patients with premature rupture of membranes at 25 to 30 weeks gestation. Am J Obstet Gynecol 1987;157:388-93.

Geirsson RT, Namunkangula R, Calder AA, Lunan CB. Preterm singleton breech presentation:the impact of traumatic intracranial haemorrhage on neonatal mortality. J Obstet Gynecol 1982;2:219-23.

Gibbs RS, Dinsmoor MJ, Newton ER, Ramamurthy RS. A randomised trial of intrapartum versus immediate postpartum treatment of women with intra-amniotic infection. Obstet Gynecol 1988;72;823-7.

Gilstrap LC, Bawdon RE, Burris J. Antibiotic concentration in maternal blood, cord blood, and placental membranes in chorioamnionitis. Obstet Gynecol 1988a;72:124-5.

Gilstrap LC, Leveno KJ, cox S, Burris JS, Mashburn M, Rosenfeld CR. Intrapartum treatment of acute chorioamnionitis: impact on neonatal sepsis. Am J Obstet Gynecol 1988b;159:579-83.

Gold V. Zentrabl Gynak 1927;24:1491.

Goldenberg RL, Nelson KG. The premature breech. Am J Obstet Gynecol 1977;127:240-4.

Gravenhorst JB, Schreuder AM, Veen S, Brand R, Verloove Vanhorick-SP, Verweij RA, van Zeben van der Aa DM, Ens Dokkum MH. Breech delivery in very preterm and very low birthweight infants in The Netherlands. Br J Obstet Gynaecol 1993;100:411-15.

Hadlock FP, Harrist RB, Carpenter RJ, Russell LD, Seung KP. Sonographic estimation of fetal weight. Radiology 1984;150:535-42.

Haesslein HC, Goodlin RC. Delivery of the Tiny newborn. Am J Obstet Gynecol 1979;134:192-200.

Harding JA, Jackson DM, Lewis DF, Major CA, Nageotte MP, Asrat T. Correlation of amniotic fluid index and nonstress test in patients with premature rupture of membranes. Am J Obstet Gynecol 1991;165:1088-94.

Harrison MR, Bressack MA, Churg AM, de Lorimer AA. Correction of congenital diaphragmatic hernia in utero. Simulated correction permits fetal lung growth with survival at birth. Surg 1980;88:260-8.

Howard TE, Killam AP, Penney LL, Daniell WC. A double blind, randomised study of terbutaline in premature labour. Milit Med 1982;147:305-7.

Iams JD, Talbert ML, Barrows H, Sachs L. Management of preterm prematurely ruptured membranes: A prospective randomised comparison of observation versus steroids and timed delivery. Am J Obstet Gynecol 1985;151:32-8.

Ingemarsson I, Westgren M, Svenningsen NW. Long term follow up of preterm infants in breech presentation delivered by caesarean section. Lancet 1978;I;172-5.

Ingemarsson I. Effect of terbutaline on premature labour. A double blind placebo controlled study. Am J Obstet Gynecol 1976;125:520-4.

Johnson JWC, Egerman RS, Moorhead J. Cases with ruptured membranes that reseal. Am J Obstet Gynecol 1990;163:1024-32.

Johnston MM, Sanchez-Ramos L, Vaughn AJ, Todd MW, Benrubi GI. Antibiotic therapy in preterm premature rupture of the membranes: A randomised, prospective, double blind trial. Am J Obstet Gynecol 1990;163:743-7.

Karp LE, Doney JR, McCarthy T, Meis PJ, Hall M. The premature breech: trial of labour or cesarean section ? Obstet Gynecol 1979;53:88-92.

Kauppila O, Gronroos M, Aro P, Aittoniemi P, Kuoppala M. management of low birh weight breech delivery: should caesarean section be routine? Obstet Gynecol 1981;57:289-94.

Kauppila O. The perinatal mortality in breech deliveries and onservations on affecting factors . Acta Obstet Gynecol Scand 1975;s39:29-35.

Kho MS, Miller JM, Brown HL, Gabert HA. Estimating tetal weight in patients with preterm premature rupture of the membranes. Am J Obstet Gynecol 1989;160:1150-4.

King AG. The determination of rupture of membranes. Am J Obstet Gynecol 1935;30:860-2.

Kitchen W, Ford GW, Doyle LW, Rickards AL, Lissenden JV, Pepperell RJ, Duke JE. Cesarean section or vaginal delivery at 24-28 weeks gestation: Comparison of survival and neonatal and two year morbidity. Obstet Gynecol 1985;66:149-57.

Kushner DH, Chang IW, Vercruysse JM. Fluorescence microscopy for determination of ruptured fetal membranes by vaginal smear. Obstet Gynecol 1964;23:196-9.

Lameier LN, Katz VL. Amnioinfusion: a review. Obstet Gynecol Surv 1993;48;12:829-36.

Lamont RF, Dunlop PDM, Crowley P, Elder MG. Spontaneous preterm labour and delivery at under 34 weeks gestation. BMJ 1983;286:454-7.

Lao TT, Halpern SH, Crosby ET, Huh C. Uterine incision and maternal blood loss in preterm caesarean section. Arch Gynecol Obstet 1993;252:113-17.

Larsen JF, Eldon K, Lange AP, Leegaard M, Osler M, Sedeberg Olsen J, Permin M. Ritodrine in the treatment of pretermm labour: second Danish multicentre study. Obstet Gynecol 1986;67:607-13.

Larsen JF, Kern HM, Hesseldahl H, Kristoffersen K, Larsen PK, Osler M, Weber J, Eldon K, Lange A. Ritodrine in the treatment of preterm labour. A clinical trial to compare a standard treatment with three regimes involving the use of ritodrine. Br J Obstet Gynaecol 1980;87:949-57.

Lawrence S, Rosenfeld CR. Fetal pulmonary development and abnormalities of amniotic fluid volume. Sem Perinat 1986;10:142-53.

Leveno KJ, Guzick DS, Hankind GDV, Klein VR, Young DC, Williams ML. Single centre randomised trial of ritodrine hydrochloride for preterm labour. Lancet 1986;I:1293-6.

Levy D, Warsof SL. Oral ritodrine and preterm premature rupture of membranes. Obstet Gynecol 1985;66:621-33.

Lewis DF, Major CA, Towers CV, Asrat T, Harding JA, Garite TJ. Effects of digital vaginal examination on latency period in preterm premature rupture of membranes. Obstet Gynecol 1992;80;630-4.

Liggins GC, Howie RN. A controlled trial of antepartum glucocorticoid treatment for the prevention of the respiratory distress syndrome in premature infants. Pediatrics 1972;50:515-25.

Liggins GC, Vilos GA, Campos GA, Kitterman JA, Lee CH. The effect of spinal cord transection on lung development in fetal sheep. J Dev Physiol 1981;3:267-74.

Lobb MO, Duthie SJ, Cooke RWI. The influence of episiotomy on the neonatal survival and incidence of periventricular haemorrhage in very low birth weight infants. Eur J Obstet Gynecol Reprod Biol 1986;22:17-21.

Lockwood CJ, Costigan K, Ghidini A, Wein R, Chien D, Brown BL, Alvarez M, Cetrulo CL. Double blind, placebo controlled trial of piperacillin prophylaxis in preterm membrane rupture. Am J Obstet Gynecol 1993;169:970-6.

Lockwood CJ, Wein R, Chien D, Ghidini A, Alvarez M, Berkowitz RL. Fetal membrane rupture is associated with the presence of insulin-like growth factor-binding protein-1 in vaginal secretions. Am J Obstet Gynecol 1994;171:146-50.

Lyons ER, Papsin FR. Cesarean section in the management of breech presentation. Am J Obstet Gynecol 1978;130:558-61.

Macri CJ, Schrimmer DB, Greenspoon JS, Strong TH, Paul RH. Amnioinfusion does not affect the length of labour. Am J Obstet Gynecol 1992;167:1134-6.

Main DM, Main EK, Maurer MM. Cesarean section versus vaginal delivery for the breech fetus weighing less than 1500 grams. Am J Obstet Gynecol 1983;146: 580-4.

Malhotra D, Gopalan S, Narang A. Preterm breech delivery in a developing country. Int J Gynaecol Obstet 1994;45:27-34.

Malloy MH, Rhoads GG, Schramm W, Land G. Increasing cesarean section rates in very low birth weight infants. Effect on outcome. JAMA 1989;262:1475-8.

Maltau JM, Egge K, Moe N. Retinal haemorrhages in the preterm neonate. A prospective randomised study comparing the occurence of haemorrhages after spontaneous versus forceps delivery. Acta Obstet Gynecol Scand 1984;63:219-21.

Mann L, Gallant JM. Modern management of the breech delivery. Am J Obstet Gynecol 1979;134:611-14.

McDuffie RS, McGregor JA, Gibbs RS. Adverse perinatal outcome and resistant enterobacteriaceae after antibiotic usage for premature rupture of the membranes and group B streptococcus carriage. Obstet Gynecol 1993;82:487-9.

McGregor JA, French JI, Reller LB, Todd JK, Makowski EL. Adjunctive erythromycin treatment for ideopathic preterm labour: Results of a randomised, double blind, placebo controlled trial. Am J Obstet Gynecol 1986;154:98-103.

McGregor JA, French JI, Seo K. Adjunctive clindamycin therapy for preterm labour: results of a double-blind, placebo-controlled trial. Am J Obstet Gynecol 1991a;165:867-75.

McGregor JA, French JI, Seo K. Antimicrobial therapy in preterm premature rupture of membranes:results of a prospective, double-blind, placebo-contolled trial of erythromycin. Am J Obstet Gynecol 1991b;165:632-40.

McGregor JA, Schoonmaker JM, Lunt BD, Lawellin DW. Antibiotic inhibition of bacterially induced fetal membrane weakening. Obstet Gynecol 1990;76:124-27.

Mercer BM, Moretti ML, Prevost RR, Sibai BM. Erythromycin therapy in preterm premature rupture of the membranes: A prospective, randomised trial of 220 patients. Am J Obstet Gynecol 1992;166:794-802.

Meyer BA, Gonik B, Creasy RK. Evaluation of phenazopyridine hydrochloride as a tool in the diagnosis of premature rupture of the membranes. Am J Perinatol 1991;8:297-9.

Milwidsky A, Finci-Yeheskel Z, Mayer M. Direct inhibition of proteases and cervical plasminogen activator by antibiotics. Am J Obstet Gynecol 1992;166:606-12.

Moberg LJ, Garite TJ, Freeman RK. Fetal heart rate patterns and fetal distress in patients with preterm premature rupture of membranes. Obstet Gynecol 1984;64:60-4.

Moessinger AC, Higgins A, Fox HE, Rey HR. Fetal breathing movements are not a reliable predictor of continued lung development in pregnancies complicated by oligohydramnios. Lancet 1987;ii:1297-9.

Morales WJ, Angel GL, O'Brien WF, Knuppel RA, Finazzo M. A randomised study of antibiotic therapy in idiopathic preterm labour. Obstet Gynecol 1988;72:829-33.

Morales WJ, Angel JL, O'Brien WF, Knuppel RA. Use of ampicillin and corticosteroids in premature rupture of membranes: A randomised study. Obstet Gynecol 1989;73:721-6.

Morales WJ, Diebel ND, Lazar AJ, Zadrozny D. The effect of antenatal dexamethasone administration on the prevention of respiratory distress syndrome in preterm gestations with premature rupture of membranes. Am J Obstet Gynecol 1986a;154:591-5.

Morales WJ, Koerten J. Obstetric management and intraventricular haemorrhage in very low birth weight infants. Obstet Gynecol 1986;68:35-40.

Morrison JC, Whtbrew WD, Bucovaz ET, Schneider JM. Injection of corticosteroids into mother to prevent neonatal respiratory distress syndrome. Am J Obstet Gynecol 1978;134:358-66.

Munson LA, Graham A, Koos BJ, Valenzuela GJ. Is there a need for digital examination in patients with spontaneous rupture of membranes. Am J Obstet Gynecol 1985;153:562-3.

Nageotte MP, Freeman RK, Garite TJ, Dorchester W. Prophylactic intrapartum amnioinfusion inpatients with premature rupture of membranes. Am J Obstet Gynecol 1985;153:557-62.

Nakayama PK, Glick PL, Harrison, Villa RL, Noall R. Experimental pulmonary hypoplasia due to oligohydramnios and its reversal by relieving thoracic compression. J Pediatr Surg 1983;18:347-53.

Nelson LH, Meis PJ, Hatjis CG, Ernest JM, Dillard R, Schey HM. Premature rupture of membranes: A prospective, randomised evaluation of steroids, latent phase, and expectant management. Obstet Gynecol 1985;66:55-8.

Newton ER, Dinsmoor MJ, Gibbs RS. A randomised, blinded, placebo controlled trial of antibiotics in idiopathic preterm labour. Obstet Gynecol 1989;74:562-7.

Newton ER, Shields L, Ridgway LE, Berkus MD, Elliot BD. Combination antibiotics and indomethacin in idiopathic preterm labour: A randomised double blind clinical trial. Am J Obstet Gynecol 1991;165:1753-9.

Nicolini U, Fisk NM, Rodeck CH, Talbert DG, Wigglesworth JS. Low amniotic pressure in oligohydramnios – is this the cause of pulmonary hypoplasia? Am J Obstet Gynecol 1989;161:1098-101.

Norman K, Pattinson RC, DeSouza J, DeJong P, Moller G, Kirsten G. Ampicillin and metronidazole treatment in preterm labour: a multicentre, randomised controlled trial. Br J Obstet Gynaecol 1994;101:404-8.

Ogita S, Imanaka M, Matsumoto M, Oka T, Sugawa T. Transcervical amnioinfusion of antibiotics: A basic study for managing premature rupture of membranes. Am J Obstet Gynecol 1988a;158:23-7.

Ogita S, Mizuno M, Takeda Y, Arai M, Sugawa T, Kuwabara y, Hashimoto T, Nishijima M, Imanaka M. Clinical effectiveness of a new cervical indwelling catheter in the management of premature rupture of the membranes: a Japanese collaborative study. Am J Obstet Gynecol 1988b;159:336-41.

Ohlsson A, Fong K, Hannah M. Prediction of lethal pulmonary hypoplasia and chorioamnionitis by assessment of fetal breathing. Br J Obstet Gynaecol 1991;98:692-7.

Olshan AF, Shy KK, Luthy DA, Hickok D, Weiss NS, Daling JR. Cesarean birth and neonatal mortality in very low birth weight infants. Obstet Gynecol 1984;64:267-70.

Owen J, Groome LJ, Hauth JC. Randomised trial of prophylactic antibiotic therapy after preterm amnion rupture. Am J Obstet Gynecol 1993;169:976-81.

Paavola A. Methods based on the study of crystals and fat staining: Use in diagnosing rupture of the membranes. Ann Chir Gynaecol Fenn 1958;47:22-8.

Papageorgiou AN, Desgranges MF, Masson M, Colle E, Shatz R, Gelfand MM. The antenatal use of betamethasone in the prevention of respiratory distress syndrome. A controlled double blind study. Pediatrics 1979;63:73-9.

Penn ZJ, Steer PJ. How obstetricians manage the problem of preterm delivery with special reference to the preterm breech. Br J Obstet Gynaecol 1991; 98: 531-34.

Philip AG, Allan WC. Does cesarean section protect against intraventricular hemorrhage in preterm infants? J Perinatol 1991;11:3-9.

Poore ER, Walker DR. Chest wall movements during fetal breathing in the sheep. J Physiol 1980;301:307-15.

Roberts AB, Mitchell JM. Direct ultrasonographic measurement of fetal lung length in normal pregnancies and pregnancies complicated by prolonged rupture of membranes. Am J Obstet Gynecol 1990;163:1560-6.

Rochelson BL, Rodke G, White R, Bracero L, Baker DA. A rapid colorimetric AFP monoclonal antibody test for the diagnosis of preterm rupture of the membranes. Obstet Gynecol 1987;69:163-7.

Romero R, Sibai B, Caritis S, Paul R, Depp R, Rosen M, Klebanoff M, Sabo V, Evans J, Thom E, Cefalo R, McNellis D. Antibiotic treatment of preterm labour with intact membranes: A multicenter, randomised, double-blinded, placebo-controlled trial. Am J Obstet Gynecol 1993;169:764-74.

Rosen RG, Chik L. The effect of delivery route on outcome in breech presentation. Am J Obstet Gynecol 1984;148:909-14.

Rotschild A, Ling EW, Puterman ML, Farquharson D. Neonatal outcome after prolonged preterm rupture of the membranes. Am J Obstet Gynecol 1990;162:46-52.

Schmidt PL, Simms ME, Strassner HT, Paul RH, Mueller E, McCart D. Effect of antepartum glucocorticoid administration upon neonatal respiratory distress syndrome and perinatal infection. Am J Obstet Gynecol 1984;148:178-86.

Schutte MF, Treffers PE, Koppe JG, Breur W, Filedt KoK JC. The clinical use of corticosteroids for acceleration of foetal lung maturity. Ned Tijdschr Geneeskd 1979;123:420-7.

Schwartz DB, Miodovnik M, Lavin JP. Neonatal outcome amnong low birth weight infants delivered spontaneously or by low forceps. Obstet Gynecol 1983;62:283-6.

Shepard MJ, Richards VA, Berkowitz RL, Warsof SL, Hobbins JC. An evaluation of two equations for predicting fetal weight by ultrasound. Am J Obstet Gynecol 1982;142:47-54.

Silver RK, MacGregor SN, Hobart ED. Impact of residual amniotic fluid volume in patients receiving parenteral tocolysis after premature rupture of the membranes. Am J Obstet Gynecol 1989;161:784-87.

Smith RP. A technic for the detection of rupture of the membranes. Obstet Gynecol 1976;48:172-6.

Sorenson T, Hasch E, Lange AP. Fetal presentation during pregnancy. Lancet 1979;ii:477

Spellacy WN, Cruz AC, Birk SA, Buhi WC. Treatment of premature labour with ritodrine: a randomised controlled study. Obstet Gynecol 1979;54:220-3.

Sperling RS, Ramamurthyr S, Gibbs S. A comparison of intrapartum versus immediate postpartum treatment of intraamniotic infection. Obstet Gynecol.1987;70:861-4.

Taeusch HW, Frigoletto F, Kitzmiller J, Avery ME, Hehre A, Fromm B, Lawson E, Neff RK. Risk of respiratory distress syndrome after prenatal dexamethasone treatment. Pediatrics 1979;63:64-72.

Teramo K, Hallman M, Raivio KO. Maternal glucocorticoid in unplanned premature labour. Pediatr Res 1980;14:326-9.

Toohey JS, Lewis DF, Harding JA, crade M, Asrat T, Major CA, Garite TJ, Porto M. Does amniotic fluid index affect the accuracy of estimated fetal weight in preterm premature rupture of membranes? Am J Obstet Gynecol 1991;165:1060-2.

Valea FA, Watson WJ, Seeds JW. Accuracy of ultasonic weight prediction in the fetus with preterm premature rupture of membranes. Obstet Gynecol 1990;75:183-4.

Van Eyck J, van der Mooren K, Wladimiroff JW. Ductus arteriosus flow velocity modulation by fetal breathing movements as a measure of fetal lung development. Am J Obstet Gynecol 1990;163:558-66.

Vergani P, Ghidini A, Locatelli A *et al*. Risk factors for pulmonary hypoplasia in second-trimester premature rupture of membranes. Am J Obstet Gynecol 1994;170:1359-64.

Volet B, Morier-Genoud J. The crystallisation test in amniotic fluid. Gynaecologia 1960;149:151-61.

Von Numers C. A new method of diagnosis of rupture of the membranes. Acta Obstet Gynecol Scand 1936;16:249-60.

Weiner CP, Renk K, Klugman M. The therapeutic efficacy and cost effectiveness of aggressive tocolysis for premature labour associated with premature rupture of the membranes. Am J Obstet Gynecol 1988;159:216-22.

Wigglesworth JS, Desai R, Guerrini P. Fetal lung hypoplasia: Biochemical and structural variations and their possible significance. Arch Dis Child 1981;56: 606-15.

Wigglesworth JS, Desai R. Effects on lung growth of cervical cord section in the rabbit fetus. Early Hum Dev 1979;3:51-65.

Wigglesworth JS, Winston RM, Bartlett K. Influence of the central nervous system on fetal lung development. Arch Dis Child 1977;52:965-7.

Winkler M, Baumann L, Ruckhaberle KE, Schiller EM. Erythromycin therapy for subclinical intrauterine infection in threatened preterm delivery - a preliminary report. J Perinatal Med 1988;16:253-4.

Wong GP, Farquharson DF, Dansereau J. Emergency cervical cerclage: A retrospective review of 51 cases. Am J Perinatol 1993;10;5:341-6.

Woods JR. Effects of low birth weight breech delivery on neonatal mortality. Obstet Gynecol 1979;53:735-40.

Yeast JD, Garite TR. The role of cervical cerclage in the management of preterm premature rupture of the membranes. Am J Obstet Gynecol 1988;158:106-10.

Index